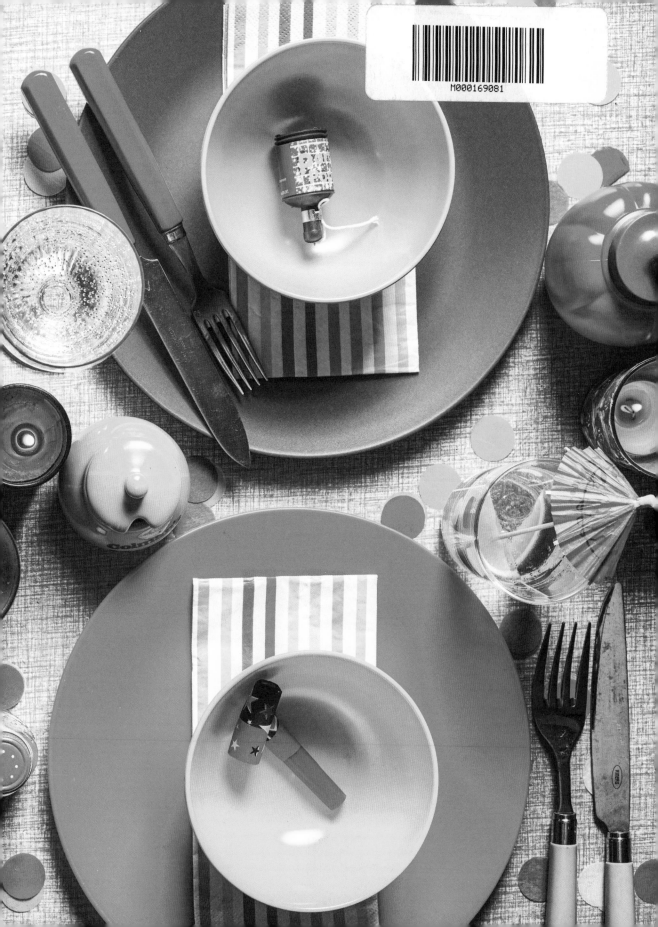

TWOCHUBBYCUBS

TWOCHUBBYCUBS
DINNER TIME

Tasty, slimming dishes for every day of the week

James Anderson & Paul Anderson

Photography by Liz and Max Haarala Hamilton

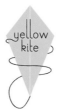

yellow
kite

First published in Great Britain in 2022 by Yellow Kite
An imprint of Hodder & Stoughton
An Hachette UK company

1

A CIP catalogue record for this title is available from the
British Library

Hardback ISBN 978 1 529 34004 4
eBook ISBN 978 1 529 340051

Colour origination by Alta Image London
Printed and bound in Germany by Mohn Media

Hodder & Stoughton policy is to use papers that are
natural, renewable and recyclable products and made
from wood grown in sustainable forests. The logging and
manufacturing processes are expected to conform to the
environmental regulations of the country of origin.

Yellow Kite
Hodder & Stoughton Ltd
Carmelite House
50 Victoria Embankment
London EC4Y 0DZ

www.yellowkitebooks.co.uk
www.hodder.co.uk

Notes

The information and references contained herein are for
informational purposes only. They are designed to
support, not replace, any ongoing medical advice given by
a healthcare professional and should not be construed as
the giving of medical advice nor relied upon as a basis for
any decision or action.

Readers should consult their doctor before altering their
diet, particularly if they are on a set diet prescribed by
their doctor or dietician.

The calorie count for each recipe is an estimate only and
may vary depending on the brand of ingredients used, and
due to the natural biological variations in the composition
of foods such as meat, fish, fruit and vegetables. It does
not include the nutritional content of garnishes or any
optional accompaniments recommended for taste/serving
in the ingredients list.

Where not specified, ingredients are analysed as average
or medium, not small or large. Eggs are medium, butter is
unsalted and milk is semi-skimmed unless otherwise
stated. All vegetables are washed.

Associate Publisher: Lauren Whelan
Project Editor: Isabel Gonzalez-Prendergast
Copy-editor: Annie Lee
Nutritionist: Kerry Torrens
Internal Design: Clare Skeats
Photographers: Liz and Max Haarala Hamilton
Food Stylist: Frankie Unsworth
Prop Stylist: Jen Kay
Production Manager: Diana Talyanina

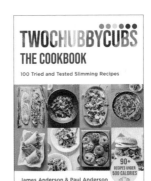

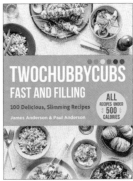

CONTENTS

INTRODUCTION

We start this book by asking you to picture a scene in your mind. Don't close your eyes, please, you'll never be able to read the description below, unless our publishers really have pushed the boat out and created an audiobook. If that's the case, I apologise in advance for my voice: if you were expecting Robson Green and got Linda Robson then I can imagine you're disappointed. Not because Linda doesn't have a lovely voice, you understand, but she isn't a 37-year-old Geordie bloke either. We digress – but do get used to that – so back to your imagination.

Imagine two *incredibly* handsome men in a stylishly equipped kitchen. One has a fabulously shaped beard and dresses like he's just wandered in from a Fred Perry photoshoot somewhere frightfully exotic. He's calm, solid and smells like the breath of a giggling angel. The other, slightly shorter, yes, but no less striking on the eye, is moving around the kitchen with the delicate grace of a ballet dancer, his deft movements belying his rotund stature.

Perhaps you'll imagine music in the background – something tasteful, non-intrusive, an LP selected at leisure from a charming retro store in a *darling* town on the shores of Lake Como. You look at the table between them, adorned with succulent treats: plates full of steamy stews, bowls of precious pastas and salads that look as though they've fallen from the gods above. The silverware gleams as the candles burn brightly and the wine – perfectly paired and poured – flows as free as a mountain brook after autumn rain.

You can hear their conversation – airy snippets of relaxed days, delivered with laughter and love. Even the silences that swell are impeccably timed. It is an image that warms your soul, gladdens your heart and makes you want to reach through the ethereality of your mind and join them for dinner.

Well, imagine all of that playing as an advert on a telly far too big for the living-room, with two slack-jawed blokes sat in front of it, both with their evening meal perched on their knees, picking half a Springer spaniel's worth of dog hair out of the mash, and you've got us: the twochubbycubs. About as fancy and elegant as a floozy behind the bins of a flat-roofed social club, us.

Speaking of us, and frankly we can think of no finer topic of conversation, a little on who we are. Long-time readers of the blog and the books will already know, but for those tight buggers who have been holding out until our books appeared in charity shops or the bargain bin at Asda, an update. I am James: six foot two and a smile that lights up a room. It's like the lights on a crashing plane, only the exit you'll be guided towards will always be behind me. Oh, behave. I'm the writer and it is my job to fill every other sentence of our books and blogs with nonsense and words that haven't been heard since the nineteenth century. I'd blame Susie Dent, but she's precious to us all.

On that note, a note of apology: at various points in this book I will switch between writing as me and writing for the two of us as the cubs. So please forgive any stray switches of perspective and grammatical errors: I did try, we promise, but we know not what I did.

Paul, on the other slightly less fat hand, is the cook and the one (mostly!) who will disappear into the kitchen for an hour or two and then burst through the doors with something delicious for me. Sometimes he even manages to do it without setting the kitchen on fire, which comes as a blessed relief as I've only got one half-naked sprint into the garden in me per year. Paul couldn't cook to save his life when we first got together, but is now confident and sassy among his shiny saucepans – testament indeed that you can do anything you set your mind towards, even if you do need to stand on an apple-box to reach the kitchen counters.

Together we are known as the twochubbycubs – two blokes both alike in a lack of dignity who like to

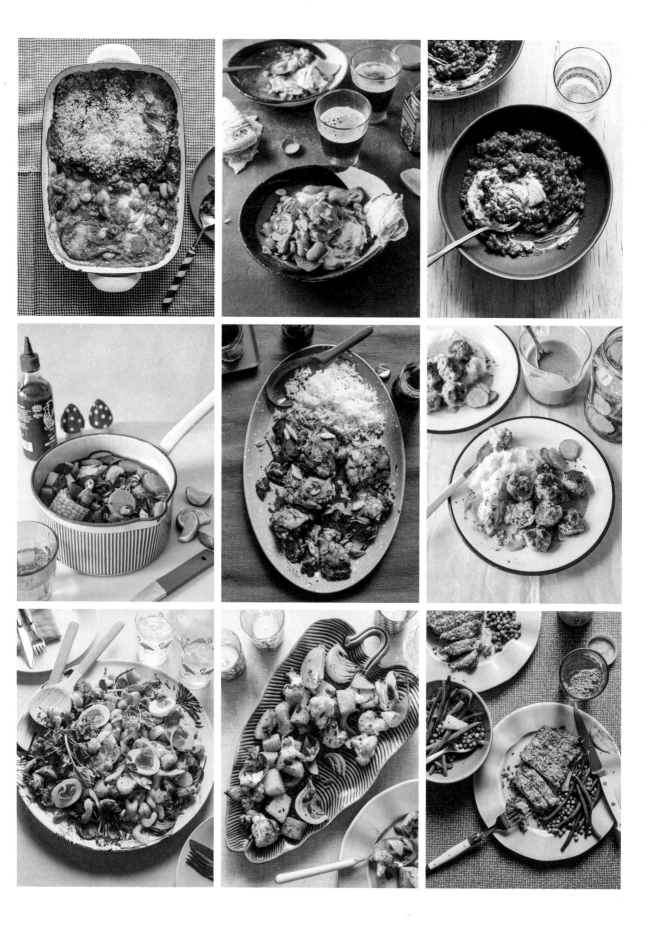

cook well, eat better and, more importantly, have fun along the way. Our blog has been running for nine years and although the title of cubs is starting to do some seriously heavy-lifting as we both advance in years and simultaneously make an 'oooh' noise when we spot a comfy chair, it's still excellent fun for us to write and cook for you all. Neither of us can believe that we've managed to convince anyone – let alone our publishers – that we are ones to follow, yet somehow we persist. You choo-choo-chose us, and we're ever so grateful.

With the blog in mind, a reminder to most and a warning to others: we don't half like to gab. You'll spot from our recipe intros that we don't focus on waffling on about some ingredient and bore you to death, but rather like to use them as jumping-off points to talk about something entirely irrelevant. We have toned down the swearing because we've spotted that some of you like to give the books to your infants as though they were rusks, but aside from that, this is just the blog in book form.

Now, we want to make one thing clear from the off, as we always do: we are not chefs. We aren't trained, we aren't food scientists, we're not nutritionists – we really are just two blokes who enjoy cooking and talking about themselves. With this in mind, we want you to know that not a single recipe in this book should cause you any difficulty when cooking, and we have kept the recipes as simple and as direct as we can. You'll be straining nothing more than excellently cooked pasta, we promise. If you're new to cooking or unsure of yourself in the kitchen, make us a promise: try the recipes you're not sure of. Give them a go: worst case scenario is that you'll have some delicious food, even if it doesn't look quite right. And for those more confident, use the recipes as a jumping-off point: the best dishes are the ones you make your own. Change the ingredients, add some extra spice – it doesn't matter as long as what you cook tickles your pickle.

With the inspiration delivered, we must now address the elephant in the room: why a book solely dedicated to evening meals?

To answer, we must first start with a confession: neither of us do breakfasts. Never have. Very occasionally we'll decide to buck our ideas up and start the day in a healthy way, but this ethos never lasts. I've long since come to terms with the fact that my morning routine will forever consist of 800 cigarettes and a can of Monster. Paul is much the same, though sometimes he'll sneak back to bed with the smell of ketchup and hash-browns on his breath.

As a result, coming up with breakfast recipes was always an utter pain – there's only so many ways you can faff about with an egg or grill some bacon before you just want to get back into bed. Don't get us wrong, we love a jar of overnight oats as much as the next person pretends to, and a fried breakfast is never going to be turned away with a haughty sneer, but for us the evening meal is the one we plan and look forward to. So, with that in mind, we wanted to create a book that you'll turn to for your most important meal – your dinner – and thus here it is.

The biggest problem when writing a book about dinner is that every single person and their dog seems to call their evening meal something different. As someone from the North East, it's tea. Paul, having been born in the wagon of a travelling show, calls it dinner. People who make their own tapenade and unironically listen to *The Archers* refer to their evening meal as supper, which is the most ludicrous of all, given supper clearly refers to the 11 p.m. dash to McDonald's because dinner didn't quite hit the spot, or in the case of my childhood, the four slices of buttered toast sprinkled with cinnamon and sugar that I used to sneak before bed. For the sake of keeping those most likely to send us 'correction' letters quiet, I've acquiesced and agreed to 'dinner' rather than 'tea'. But please, know that you're wrong.

But, when you think about it, I'm not wrong about dinner being the most important of our meals. Breakfast is nearly always a dashed affair, even when you're one of those awful American sitcom families where the harried-looking matriarch prepares a breakfast spread that spans the entire table, only for her husband to dash in, grab a slice of toast and kiss her on the cheek as he flies out. Often accompanied by a teenage daughter with a face like a slapped a*se refusing to eat and the son yelling he's 'eating out at Kimberley's' as he climbs out the window. I know! I should write for TV. If those were my kids and husband they'd be eating that bloody breakfast for four days in a row. No, breakfast is solitary and easily the worst of the meal trifecta.

Then what of the humble lunch? Well, don't get me wrong, lunch has a place. But for most, lunch is sustenance crammed into the day in whatever quick form it can take to get you through the afternoon. We add leftovers of yesterday's dinner, or we buy a meal deal and feel sad about our life choices while we choke on a sandwich. A good lunch out is restorative, of course, but far from the norm. Think to yourself of your last few memorable meals – how many of those were spent scrunched over a keyboard on your lunch-break? It is rarely lunch that we look back upon and do that whimsy-smile reserved for precious memories. However, in the spirit of giving, do know this: a lot of the dinners here will be perfect for lunch the next day.

Dinner, however, is where the action is. The dinners of our respective childhoods are wildly different, though. For me, with parents who worked odd shifts and a sister who spent most of her time throwing DVD box-sets at my mother and shouting, it was the rare opportunity to have everyone together. We weren't posh, so dinners were always consumed in the same room but at different heights: parents on the sofa, sister usually sat glowering somewhere and me lying on my belly in front of the coal fire. It was during these meals I remember finding out what everyone was up to, future holiday plans, the reasons why my mother was cross with the milkman. I imagine if you were to ask them what they remembered of me during those meals it would be my abject silence, given my tendency to wolf down my dinner lest I ever get asked to share.

Paul never had the luxury of a family sit-down, though he suggests it could be because he was upstairs 'finding himself' most of the time. His mother never called him down for whatever ready-meal-delight she had hauled from the freezer that evening, though even now he sits bolt upright at the ding of a microwave. He's Pavlov's dog reborn as a human and clad in Blue Harbour seconds. He does remember, on the rare occasion of dining together, all the meals being served up on hideously patterned trays with padding underneath, presumably because his mother needed somewhere to balance her ashtray between forkfuls. We laugh about it now, but you have no idea how much use we get out of those trays these days: it's second only to having my dessert served directly from a trolley as my favourite delivery mechanism.

Nowadays, we nearly always eat together – out of necessity to a degree because lord knows I'm not going to cook when I have Paul, who I can holler at and icily criticise his offerings, but mostly out of the comfort of sitting together and blathering on to one another. Our dinners are always punctuated by some random TV because I hear screams in silence, but it's always an opportunity to catch up with one another and put the world to rights. It's telling indeed that whenever Paul goes away, even though I *can* cook, I don't bother: it's not the same without his monologues about what has vexed him or the anxiety of me watching exactly how much of his meal he's going to drop on to the carpet. That's less of an issue now thanks to the addition of Goomba, our new dog, who treats the floor like

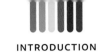

a grazing table at all times. It's also lucky that fourteen years of Paul staring at me with doleful, pleading eyes for the scraps off my plate has prepared me for the same from Goomba.

So that's why this book is exclusively dinners: because we consider them to be the most important of all. If we're wrong we apologise, and recommend you turn to our blog and previous books for breakfast and lunch ideas: you'll find some absolute blinders among the filth. But if you have come this far into the book, we'll ask you to come a little further, then laugh because we said come twice: join us for dinner!

(Elbows off the table please and I think that's your nipple in the gravy, you saucy minx.)

James & Paul x

AND FOLKS, THE CALORIES ON EACH RECIPE ARE PER PORTION!

KEEP IN TOUCH AND TAG US WITH YOUR TASTY DINNERS!

 twochubbycubs   @twochubbycubs   #twochubbycubs

HOW TO USE THE BOOK — SOME HANDY SYMBOLS:

Like in our last book, we have marked on each recipe with our handy set of symbols to streamline your cooking needs.

Over 30 minutes	Easy to scale	V Vegetarian
Under 30 minutes	Under 10 ingredients	GF Gluten-free
Freezes well	Blog recipe	DF Dairy-free

A NOTE ON BODY POSITIVITY
AND WEIGHT LOSS

You see, running a weight-loss/slimming/kn*b-joke-factory blog is a bit of a double-edged sword. We want to help people lose weight with delicious, easy-to-cook recipes that don't taste like diet food, but we also never want anyone to feel they *have* to lose weight to be happy. You don't.

Over the years, we have learned that it isn't your body that shapes your mood, but rather, how you view it. We place so much emphasis on what others think when their eyes fall upon our body – we fret about stretchmarks and the fact our nipples tickle our ears when we lie on our back and to what end?

Take me (James). I have spent about 30 of the 37 years of my life worrying about different parts of my body. I've been too fat, too thin, too tall, too short. I think I have weirdly bulgy eyes when I concentrate. I have enough forehead that I could advertise the blog on there and include all the pop-up adverts. Just when I think I've come to terms with one aspect of my body, another one demands I criticise it.

However, I am also a realist. So a few years ago, fuelled by the TV show we did, I finally took control of the one thing I could change: my weight. I figured that if I lost the weight and became thin and capable of walking into a high-street clothes shop without a collective gasp of fright, I'd be a happy man. Ten stone weight loss later: I wasn't. I don't suit being that thin – I look like a hot-air balloon crushed into a telephone mast. Physically, being that skinny wasn't for me (and note that I was still four stone away from my 'correct' weight according to my BMI, which shows what a load of tut that barometer can be) but mentally, I was so sure I'd be content at that point.

I had a period of self-reflection and I wish I could give you some epiphany here, but it's as simple as this: happiness comes from within. If you can't accept who you are, come to terms with your faults and wrinkles, you'll never be at peace.

So, how to change the outlook of someone who has spent a life criticising himself? Surprisingly easy. I stopped giving a toss about what those I didn't know thought and learned to accept the kind words of those that matter. Paul, for example, has inexplicably chosen to spend a third of his life with me and still looks happy when I come galumphing across the lawn. That ripples across my family, friends, conquests. If you ever want a good measure of yourself, take note at how those who love you look at you. Everyone else? They can eff off. Can you remember one single stranger you saw yesterday? If they're that fleeting in your life, why waste your energy worrying about what they think?

It takes time, because all good things do, but you'll realise that you're less self-critical. I actually ended up putting four stone back on, and I can say, with my hand on my heart and the other hand in a bag of crisps, I'm possibly the most content I've been with my body. Those who love me, love me, and for the first time in forever, I include myself in that.

Blimey. Feels like I've just spent an hour in the confession box. But see, I mention all of the above because sometimes it helps to hear that the confident, brassy tart behind the social media posts struggles with his body in much the same way as almost everyone else does. In being as open as I can be, I hope to help you make sure you're losing weight for the right reasons. If you want to be healthier, great, if you want to lose weight so you can get nicer clothes or play with your children, more power to your elbow. But if you're thinking you'll be happy if only you were skinnier, examine whether that's really true. We can offer you delicious food and some laughs along the way but your happiness has to come from yourself. If you use this book to lose some weight and work on your body confidence, we promise the end result will be so much more glorious.

THE ONE-POUND-A-WEEK WEIGHT LOSS CHALLENGE

Let's turn to the business of actually losing weight and the other message we push: the one-pound-a-week approach. Over the page you'll see a collection of circles, and although you may be clutching your pearls and thinking we've had a fit of the vapours (a fair enough assumption), we shall talk you through it all and encourage you to give it a go.

Both Paul and I spent years attending slimming clubs in the 'battle' to try and lose weight. Every week we would turn up, pay our subs, stand on the scales, make small-talk, then sit down and listen to everyone talk loudly about their weight losses and gains and bowel movements. I've genuinely never heard so many people talk so freely about their poops, and I used to be a medical secretary for a gastroenterologist.

The classes worked – perhaps it was the fear of stepping on the scales, perhaps it was the fact we're suckers for stickers – but the weight loss never stuck with us. We would lose a stone, maybe two, and then we would have a blip or a weight gain and that would be it: binge eating, shame-stuffing, trips to the chippy and tears of pure gravy. We completed the join up, lose weight, put weight on, stop going, rejoin cycle so many times that the church hosting the classes gave us our own parking space. We had to change the way we did things.

Now, before we get to the good bit, we want to make it clear that the above may not be your experience and that's absolutely fine – slimming classes are a good fit for some people, and if they push you to success, you must keep going and enjoy it because a successful programme is one that works for you. There's no diet shaming with twochubbycubs, unless you're taking weight-loss miracle products you bought off a sentient set of eyelashes on Facebook.

So, why didn't the weight loss stick? Why were we consistently getting a stone or two off and then not so much falling off the horse as tumbling off and

making a ragù from it? Simple: the pressure to lose four or five pounds a week. We had come to accept that such weight loss was healthy and consistently achievable, and it just isn't. As the good doctor Ian Malcolm once said, life finds a way. There will be weeks when you have plans, or when you over-eat, and sometimes you'll do everything right and for whatever reason your body is spiteful and holds on to every little morsel of fat it can, and you'll gain weight. That is life.

But if you have set yourself up to expect a few pounds a week in weight loss, then what do you feel when you've gained, stayed the same or only lost a pound or two? Angry. Upset. Ready to eat your feelings. When, of course, that's absolute and utter nonsense and it's this mentality that you need to change.

The one-pound-a-week challenge, then. It's all about reframing your approach so that you concentrate on a tiny, easily achievable target and celebrating those victories as and when they come. If you were setting out to climb a mountain, we have to presume that (after checking first to see if there was a taxi service or cable-car) you wouldn't look to sprint right to the top without resting your legs a few times on the way up. That applies to weight loss too: whether you've got three stone to lose or twenty, if you focus on one tiny target at a time, it'll feel far more do-able.

Consistently hitting your one-pound-a-week target and celebrating these tiny steps will have a happy side-effect, we guarantee: very often you'll end up losing more than a pound. The fact you're in a positive frame of mind and approaching your weight loss with no pressure on yourself will lend itself to smart decisions and guilt-free eating, which will in turn lead to bigger results on the scales. Great! But you don't record that, at least not on the chart. You stay focused on that one pound a week and everything else is a happy accident.

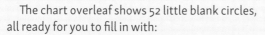

The chart overleaf shows 52 little blank circles, all ready for you to fill in with:

- a charming green if you've hit your one-pound-a-week target;
- a urine-sample yellow if you've stayed the same; and
- a raging red if you've put on weight.

If you put on weight, no belly-aching – as we said before, it'll happen and that's life. If you manage to get through the year and that chart is entirely green that's great, but we encourage you to enjoy life a little more. Weight gain shouldn't be used as a stick to beat yourself with, not least because if you're anything like us, you'll probably use a baguette.

For every few green dots you manage to complete, bloody well celebrate them. How quick we are to make a thing about our failures and yet when we have cause to celebrate, we downplay it, we don't make a fuss. That's the second thing that needs to stop: we're not suggesting you dash out and remortgage your house at every quarter stone, but do something that makes you happy. Doesn't need to be expensive: it can be going out somewhere new or seeing an old friend for dinner. You're making positive progress and that ought to be rewarded.

You can give yourself bonus points if you manage to tie your celebrations into things you had put off because of your weight, and it's here that we can talk about Paul, the ex-elephant in the room. See, for all that I can waffle on about my weight loss story until you push Wotsits in your ears and tell me to stop, Paul is this year's real hero. Eagle-eyed viewers may spot a substantial change between Paul's author photo from book one and the one we've used here: he's lost over eight stone. We both had a COVID scare: his was contracting it and struggling to breathe, mine was him contracting it and me having to make my own dinners. We've both suffered terribly.

Realising that he wasn't happy with himself and was at risk of causing himself a serious medical mischief, he set about losing the weight, following the one-pound-a-week challenge, though because he's hip and hi-tech he made himself a chart on his phone. For the first time in forever, his weight loss was consistent – week in, week out, more loss and a happier Paul. He celebrated his changes by doing all manner of things that he had put off because of his weight: a public swim, seeing mates he hadn't seen in years, actually buying clothes from somewhere other than the court-appearance-casual section on Jacamo.

As a loving husband, it was a delight to see him come back out of his shell. Whereas I've always been excellent at pretending all is OK when inside I'm all a-quiver, Paul wears his heart on his sleeve, and that sleeve has been dragged across his dinner plate. I saw him miserable and comfort-eating and always disappointed with himself when he slipped back into bad habits. This new Paul is back to being the fun, relatively easy-going chap who tumbled me roughly across a golf course for a hole-in-one when we first met and didn't walk with his face to the floor so he couldn't see people gawping at him. It's glorious.

We mention Paul's weight loss purely because he's the proof of the pudding: reframing the weight loss approach into a succession of little targets with every victory celebrated will lead to continued, manageable losses. For the first time in his entire life he's in control of his weight loss and sticking to it, and this could very easily be you. You could be Paul, though you'll need to get yourself equipped with eighty-seven pairs of stonewashed jeans before you can ever truly claim that title.

We wish you every success with your weight loss, we truly do. But remember: don't let it define you.

LET'S GET GOING!

WEEK 1

WEEK 2

WEEK 3

WEEK 4

WEEK 5

WEEK 6

WEEK 7

WEEK 8

WEEK 9

WEEK 10

WEEK 11

WEEK 12

WEEK 13

WEEK 14

WEEK 15

WEEK 16

WEEK 17

WEEK 18

WEEK 19

WEEK 20

WEEK 21

WEEK 22

WEEK 23

WEEK 24

WEEK 25

WEEK 26

WEEK 27

WEEK 28

WEEK 29

WEEK 30

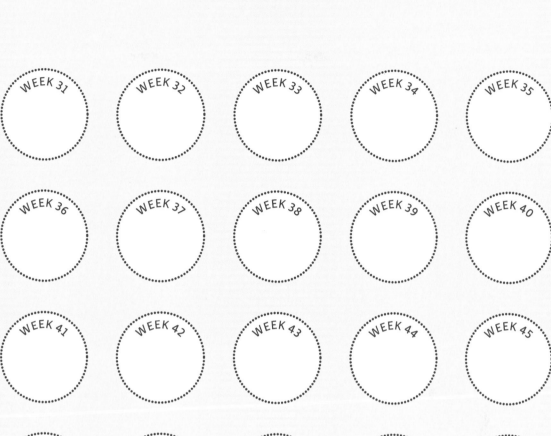

WEEK 31　WEEK 32　WEEK 33　WEEK 34　WEEK 35

WEEK 36　WEEK 37　WEEK 38　WEEK 39　WEEK 40

WEEK 41　WEEK 42　WEEK 43　WEEK 44　WEEK 45

WEEK 46　WEEK 47　WEEK 48　WEEK 49　WEEK 50

WEEK 51　WEEK 52

WE'VE HOSTED THIS DELIGHTFUL GRID ON OUR BLOG TOO, SO ONCE YOU'RE DONE – YOU CAN START OVER AND REUSE TIME AND TIME AGAIN!

30 TIPS TO HELP WITH EASY COOKING

Over the course of the last few books and years of blog-writing we have dispensed tips like nobody's business, but sometimes you need a fresh voice to give you some more inspiration. I threw the question of 'what's your favourite top tip for easy cooking' out to our Facebook followers and, once they'd stubbed out their rollies and turned the volume down on *This Morning*, they really came through. We may have paraphrased them a tad.

1. WHEN YOU'VE SELECTED A RECIPE, REMEMBER TO ACTUALLY BUY ALL THE INGREDIENTS INSTEAD OF FORGETTING THE TWO MOST CRUCIAL ONES AND THEN WONDERING WHAT BECAME OF YOUR DINNER Sarah S

2. GET A PAIR OF KITCHEN MARACAS — THEY'RE A DISTRACTION FOR OTHERS IN THE ROOM AND PROVIDE A CHARMING FIDGET TOY FOR WHEN YOU'RE STARING FURIOUSLY AT THE OVEN Gillian S

3. ALWAYS START WITH A CLEAN KITCHEN AND TIDY AS YOU GO Paul Anderson (which I've included because that man has never left a kitchen clean in his entire life, the two-faced b*stard)

4. BATCH COOK FOR THOSE NIGHTS WHEN YOU JUST CAN'T BE A*SED Heidi G

5. LEFTOVER WINE IS YOUR FRIEND, TURPENTINE LESS SO Rachel LB

6. READ EVERYTHING TWICE IN THE RECIPE — MAKE SURE YOU DON'T MISS A STEP Jenny B

7. GIVE YOUR CHILDREN A SMALL BALL OF PASTRY TO PLAY WITH WHILE YOU BAKE — MEANS YOU DON'T NEED TO EAT THE SNOT-COVERED FOOD THEY'VE 'HELPED' WITH Caroline K

8. IF YOU'RE MAKING JAMBALAYA, BE SURE TO SING IT TO THE TUNE OF BAMBOYLEO BY THE GYPSY KINGS, OTHERWISE WHAT'S THIS ALL BEEN ABOUT? Tess D

9. LISTEN TO SOMETHING YOU LOVE AS YOU COOK, SUCH AS A FUNNY AUDIOBOOK OR THE SOBBING OF THOSE YOU ENTOMBED IN THE FLOOR Claire J

10. KEEP ALL YOUR SPICES, HERBS AND OILS IN A DRAWER — IT'S ORGANISED, AND HELPS WHEN YOU'RE A SHORT-A*SE WHO CAN'T REACH THE CUPBOARD Lesley D

11. TASTE YOUR SALT WHEN YOU BUY IT — THE STRENGTH CAN CHANGE EVEN IN THE SAME BRAND, EVEN IF YOUR TONGUE IS 90% NICOTINE-LACQUERED ASBESTOS Paul H

12. USE A TROUSER HANGER WITH CLIPS AS A RECIPE BOOK HOLDER — HANG IT FROM A CUPBOARD TO GIVE MORE ROOM ON THE WORKTOP Cat D

13. IT'S NOT TIME TO MAKE A CHANGE, JUST RELAX, TAKE IT EASY, YOU'RE STILL YOUNG, THAT'S YOUR FAULT, THERE'S SO MUCH YOU HAVE TO KNOW Cat S

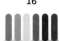

14. WRITE ON YOUR COOKBOOK WITH ANY CHANGES OR ADDITIONS THAT YOU MADE — MAKE THE RECIPE YOUR OWN   James A

15. EMBRACE SPEEDY FIXES LIKE CHOPPED VEGETABLES, FROZEN ONIONS AND JARRED GARLIC — TIME-SAVING AND CHEAP   Dawn H

16. TREAT THE COOKING EXPERIENCE AS A CATCH-UP FOR YOURSELF: READ THE RECIPE, RESEARCH THE INGREDIENTS, ENJOY THE TIME SPENT COOKING — COOKING SHOULD BE FUN, NOT A CHORE   Methuselah H

17. TASTE AS YOU GO, NOT AT THE END — EASY TO CORRECT AS YOU COOK RATHER THAN LAMENT AS YOU EAT   Lynsey R

18. TAKE YOUR TROUSERS OFF BEFORE COOKING — IT'S VERY FREEING AND WILL MAKE YOU FEEL AT ONE WITH NATURE   Toni H

20. PRACTISE, PRACTISE, PRACTISE: THINGS MAY NOT ALWAYS GO SMOOTHLY, BUT THAT'S JUST FINE   Jana J

21. TEACH YOUR KIDS TO COOK — THEY'RE FABULOUSLY FREE HELP, UNLESS THEY'RE RUBBISH OF COURSE   Lorelei S

19. DON'T STRESS ABOUT EXACT INGREDIENTS AND COOK LIKE NO ONE IS WATCHING, UNLESS YOU'VE GOT A PEEPING TOM FETISH, IN WHICH CASE MAKE SURE YOU BOIL WASH THAT ROLLING PIN   Poppy S

22. BE SURE TO TELL EVERYONE WHAT AMAZING WONDERS JAMES AND PAUL ARE, FORCE THEM TO BUY EXTRA COPIES OF THE COOKBOOK AND DON'T FORGET TO MENTION HOW MODEST, HANDSOME AND FRAGRANT JAMES IS   Jim V

23. TO MAKE SUPER CRISPY ROASTIES (THOUGH YOU DO RISK SIGNIFICANT ANGRY NOSTRIL-BREATHING FROM THE AUTHOR OF EMOTIONAL SUPPORT POTATOES), SPRINKLE WITH A BIT OF BAKING POWDER AFTER THEY'VE BEEN RUFFLED UP AND BEFORE THEY GO INTO THE HOT OIL   Karen Y

24. MAKE SURE AS MUCH AS POSSIBLE OF YOUR DINNER, COOKING, SHOES, KITCHEN EQUIPMENT, MATCHES, BOOKS, CASH AND ANYTHING IMPORTANT LANDS ON THE FLOOR SO I HAVE SOMETHING TO CHEW ON IN THOSE EIGHT SECONDS A DAY YOU DON'T HAVE YOUR EYE ON ME   Goomba A

25. BE VERSATILE IN THE KITCHEN   Jonathan A

26. I'LL BE VERSATILE WHEN I WANT TO BE, THANK YOU, SO DON'T PRESSURE ME   James Anderson

27. MAKE UP YOUR OWN SPICE MIXES — IF YOU'RE REGULARLY PULLING TOGETHER MIXES FOR A RECIPE YOU LOVE, MAKE BIG BATCHES OF THE MIX AND KEEP IT IN AIRTIGHT JARS   Helen K

28. COOK LIKE YOU'RE NIGELLA, EVEN IF YOU'RE MORE OF A FANNY   Mark L-G

29. DON'T EVER EXPECT YOUR MEALS TO LOOK LIKE THEY DO IN THE BOOK (YES — JAMES) BECAUSE THOSE PHOTOS ARE THE RESULT OF A TEAM OF STYLISTS MAKING THEM LOOK PERFECT. FOOD DOESN'T NEED TO BE INSTAGRAM PERFECT   Dominique E

30. GL 45-YEAR-OLD SINGLE WLTM COMPANION FOR GT. MUST HAVE OWN CAR, TEETH   Susan M

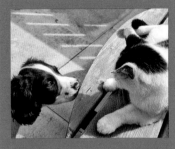

Dog and cat relations going well

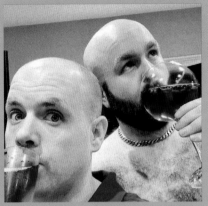

Everything in moderation

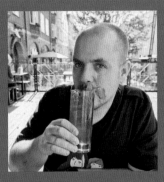

Fruity and tart, Paul enjoys a drink

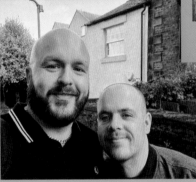

Hot single Dads in your area
(should be careful, we're about)

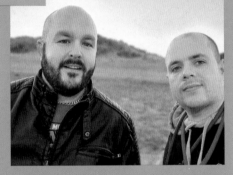

Christmas on glamorous Blyth beach

Taken in a public bathroom (so was the photo)

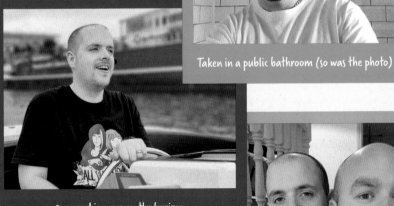

One working eye on the horizon

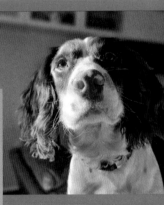

We'll have no trouble here

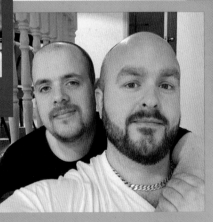

Paul had to stand on a step so we were level

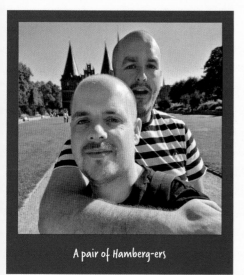

A pair of Hamberg-ers

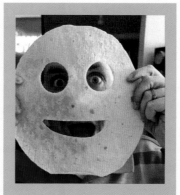

Paul's never looked more delicious

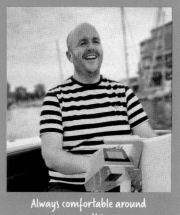

Always comfortable around seamen, this one

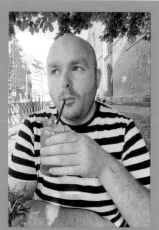

Bitter and harsh on the throat, James enjoys a drink

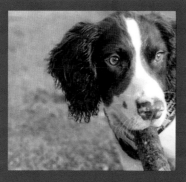

Goomba's been in James's humidor again

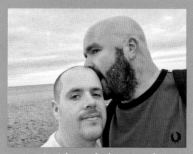

Here Paul demonstrates a second use as James's salt-lick

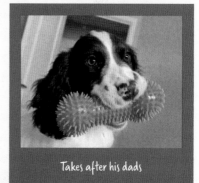

Takes after his dads

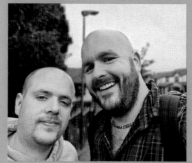

Happy faces for someone with a street-light growing from his head

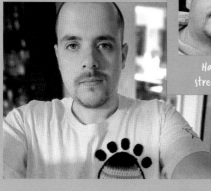

We get it Paul, you're skinny now

And Goomba makes three

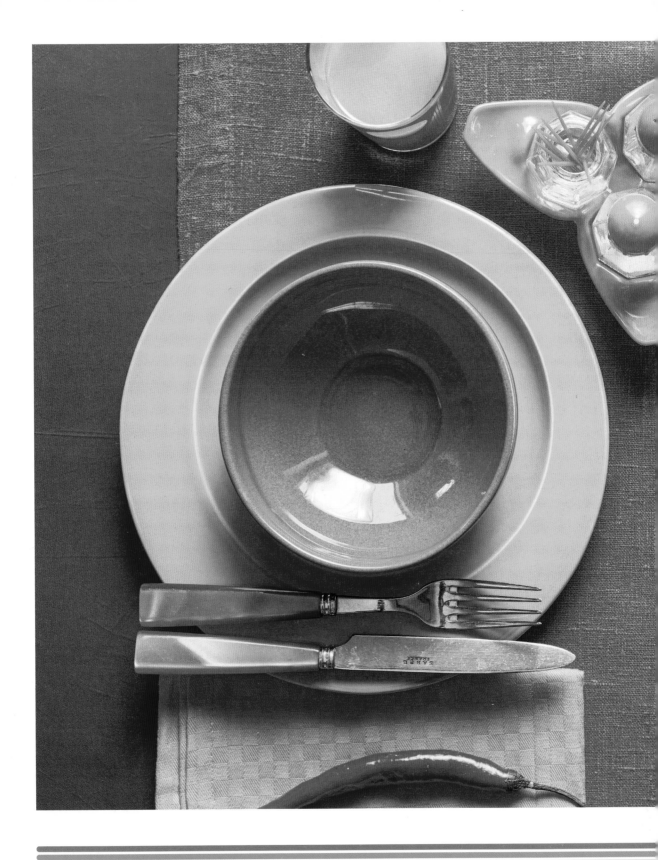

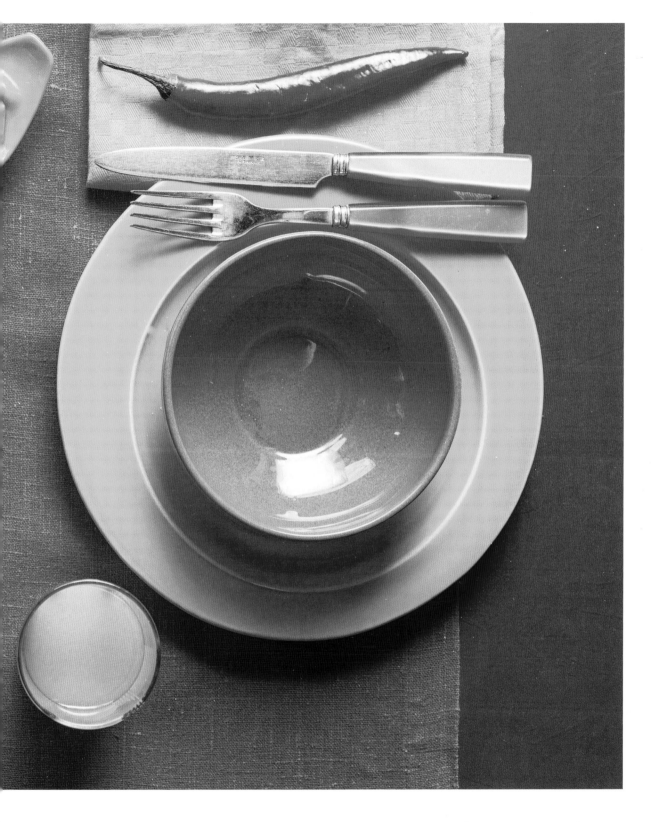

VEG & FISH

TOMATO TARTE TATIN

Tomatoes are wonderful little things, aren't they? Paul disagrees, but he does love to be contrary, unless I point out such behaviour and he agrees just to prove me wrong. But if you're a fan of the squashy, seed-filled fruit, I implore you to ignore his view on tomatoes and to make this tarte Tatin as quick as you like. I'd suggest you run home, but neither Paul nor I are in a position to make any claims about running, given I run like Dr Robotnik when he gets knocked from his machines and Paul doesn't so much run as blunder at speed.

Oh, and I know we say this often, but still people persist: do not keep your tomatoes in the fridge. You keep them in a bowl on the windowsill. We've been through this.

You know, a little tip that I'm not even going to pop in the notes because frankly I don't want to overshadow my amazing tomato cutting tip: you could absolutely make smaller versions of these and use flavoured soft cheese to do it. It wouldn't be authentic, it wouldn't be rustic, but it would be oh, oh-so-tasty.

SERVES: 4
PREP: 10 minutes
COOK: 35 minutes
CALORIES: 490

375g (13oz) light puff pastry
1 teaspoon wholegrain mustard
125g (4½oz) ricotta
1 teaspoon dried mixed herbs
500g (1lb 2oz) mixed cherry
   tomatoes, halved (or normal
   ones, sliced)
100g (3½oz) reduced-fat green
   pesto
3 tablespoons grated Parmesan
   or vegetarian Italian-style hard
   cheese
a handful of basil leaves
salt and black pepper

Preheat the oven to 220°C fan/475°F/gas 8.

Roll out the pastry and place it on a large baking sheet, then fold over the edges to create a thin crust.

Mix together the mustard, ricotta and mixed herbs and spread over the pastry.

Arrange the tomato halves or slices over the pastry, overlapping if necessary. Spray with a little oil and sprinkle over a pinch of salt and pepper, then drizzle over the pesto.

Bake in the oven for 35 minutes, then remove and scatter over the grated Parmesan and the basil leaves.

Remove from the oven and slice into four slices to serve.

NOTE

To cut a load of cherry tomatoes at once, wedge them between two chopping boards and use a long knife to slice them all at once.

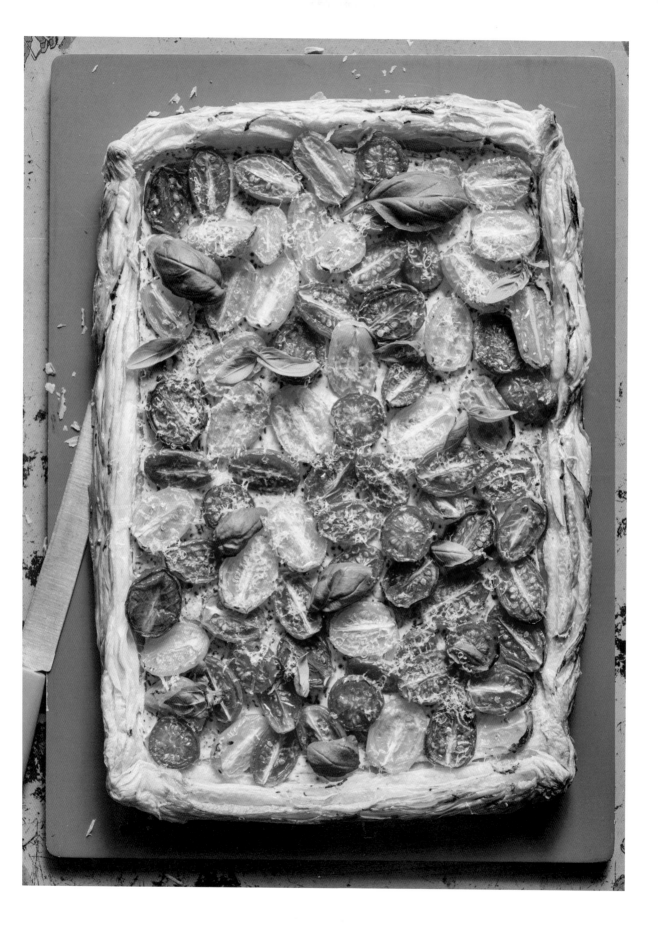

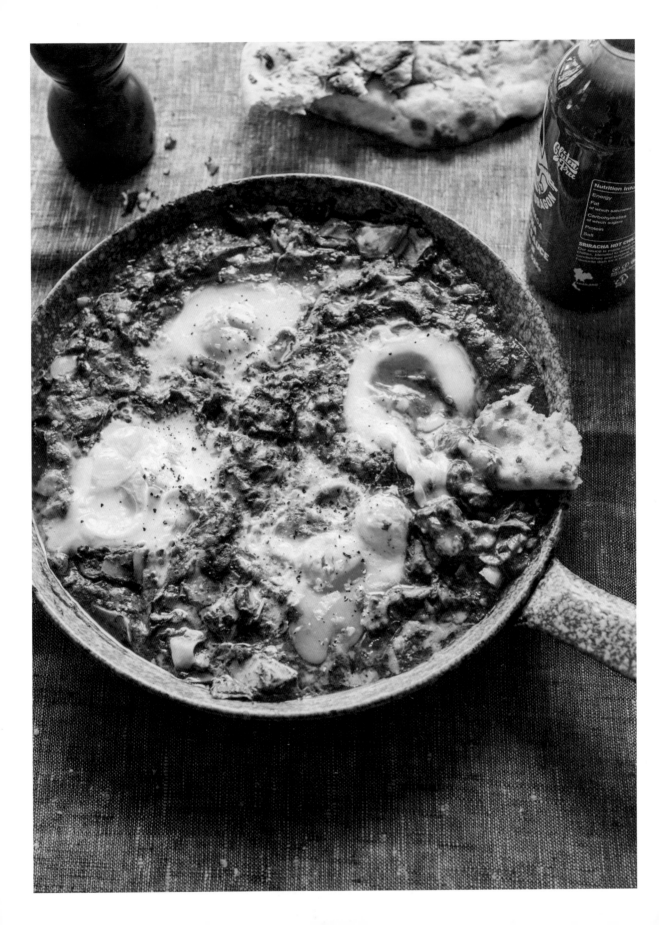

GREEN SHAKSHUKA

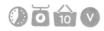

Now, here's the thing: we aren't entirely sure we can call this shakshuka because, ordinarily, that would be made with tomatoes and peppers and the like (indeed, we have a fabulous shakshuka breakfast recipe in *Fast & Filling*). So, as ever, if we have committed a cultural faux-pas, we apologise profusely: we just like this green take ever so, and anything that gets more green into you must be encouraged. Plus, this takes one of our favourite breakfast meals and turns it into something entirely different: do give it a go.

Oh, and if you happen to serve this atop buttered doorstep slices of bread or flatbreads, we won't tell a soul.

SERVES: 4
PREP: 15 minutes
COOK: 25 minutes
CALORIES: 260

3 leeks
250g (9oz) baby spinach
30g (1oz) flat-leaf parsley
70g (2½oz) low-fat soft cheese
350g (12oz) artichoke hearts, drained and chopped
40g Parmesan or vegetarian Italian-style hard cheese, grated
4 eggs
salt and black pepper

Wash the leeks and halve lengthways, then cut into 1cm (½ inch) slices.

Spray a large frying pan with a little oil and place over a medium heat. Add the leeks and cook for about 15 minutes, until soft, then remove from the heat.

Bring a saucepan of water to the boil. Add the spinach and parsley and blanch for 15 seconds, then drain in a sieve. Use a bowl to push down on the spinach and squeeze out as much liquid as possible.

Put the leeks, spinach, parsley, soft cheese and 6 tablespoons of water into a blender (or use a stick blender) and blitz until smooth.

Place the frying pan back over a medium heat and spray with a little oil. Add the artichokes and heat for about 3 minutes, stirring frequently. Add the spinach to the pan and spread out.

Sprinkle in the Parmesan and make four wells with the back of a spoon. Break an egg into each of the wells, sprinkle with a little salt and pepper and cook for 4–5 minutes.

Divide between bowls, and serve.

BLOODY RISOTTO

Take our hand for a moment and step back in time to a few years ago. Calvin Harris's 'One Kiss' was everywhere. Eileen was being terrorised by Phelan in *Corrie*, the lucky, lucky soul. Meghan married Harry, the lucky, lucky soul. And you'd find Paul and I more willing to eat fresh soil than try beetroot. And look, it makes sense: beetroot tastes like earth.

However, a chance meal in some restaurant where the menu didn't come with a pack of crayons to keep the kids occupied changed our mind. Beetroot, when baked and softened, becomes a whole new taste and, when thrown into a gentle risotto as below and masked with some goat's cheese, is really quite wonderful. Those who have been with us from the start know we are fans of the risnotto – throw it all in and gently simmer – but not here. This is one of those rare risotto recipes where you'll need to take your time to reap the rewards. I mean, as W. H. Davies definitely meant to say, 'a poor life this if, full of care, we have no time to stand and stir'. Well, kinda works. If you talk like Cilla Black. Shush, eat your risotto.

SERVES: 4
PREP: 20 minutes
COOK: 1 hour 30 minutes
CALORIES: 498

500g (1lb 2oz) fresh beetroots
80g (3oz) soft goat's cheese
1 teaspoon orange zest
2 tablespoons milk
2 onions, diced
4 cloves of garlic, crushed
   or grated
250g (9oz) Arborio rice
200ml (7fl oz) white wine
1 litre (1¾ pints) vegetable stock
1 tablespoon butter
30g (1oz) Parmesan or vegetarian
   Italian-style hard cheese,
   grated

NOTES

Bit of a clart on, but we promise it's worth it.

Don't like goat's cheese? Soft cheese like Philadelphia is fine!

Preheat the oven to 180°C fan/400°F/gas mark 6.

Wash the beetroots and remove the leaves and stalks, but don't peel! Place on a baking tray, cover with foil, and bake for 1 hour. After an hour, check they are cooked – you want to be able to push a fork through without too much pressure. If they're not quite ready, cook for another 15 minutes and try again.

Once tender, leave to cool, then peel. Roughly dice the beetroots and blend until smooth, then set aside.

Mix together the soft goat's cheese, orange zest and milk in a bowl, then set aside.

Place a large, shallow pan over a medium-high heat and spray with a little oil. Add the onions and cook for 7–8 minutes, until softened. Add the garlic and cook for a further minute. Add the rice to the pan and stir for a minute or two, until the edges of the grains are turning translucent, then pour in the wine and stir.

Add 6 tablespoons of the blended beetroot mix to the pan and stir well. Add a ladle of vegetable stock and keep stirring until it is all absorbed. Repeat this with the rest of the stock.

Remove the pan from the heat, add the butter and Parmesan, and stir well.

Serve the risotto in bowls and spoon the goat's cheese on top.

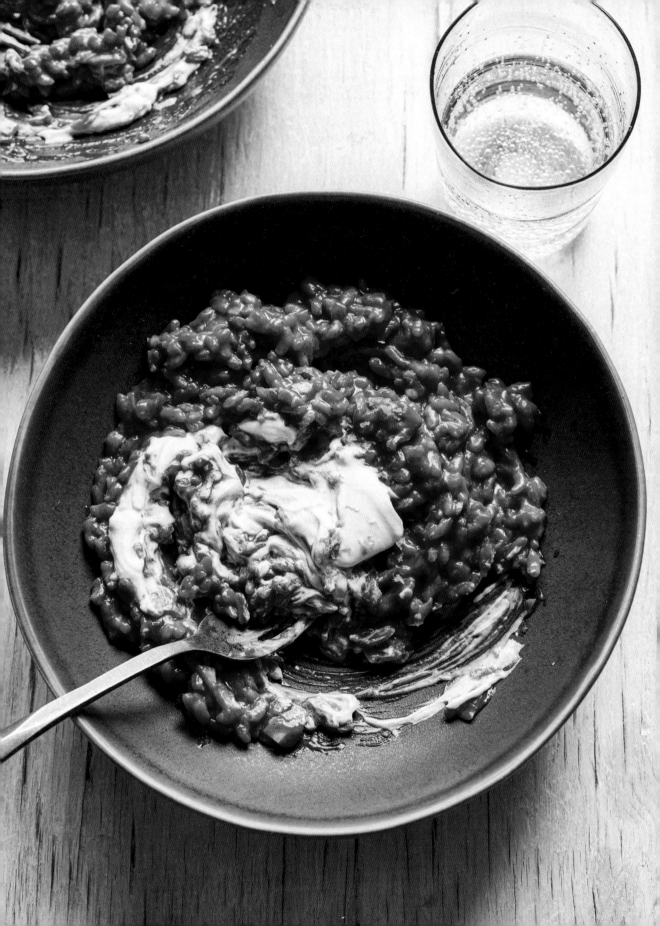

GARLIC CHEESY CHIPS

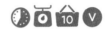

We always try to include a spin on a chips recipe in our books because sometimes it's what you need when you stumble home, hair full of the day and a face like a smacked a*se. As this is a recipe book we have made it a bit more fancy, but it's worth the farting about, I promise you. So you'll see below, although this is 'chips', it's also got leeks and all that in it.

While these are delicious, cheesy chips from a takeaway place that hides its food-hygiene scores behind its menus stuck on the door is my go-to meal when we're out on the pop. Paul prefers a cheeseburger which has never seen actual cheese or indeed, actual meat, but as long as he gets most of it down his new shirt, we're laughing.

SERVES: 4
PREP: 10 minutes
COOK: 1 hour 10 minutes
CALORIES: 499

1 tablespoon butter
2 leeks, trimmed and thinly sliced
6 cloves of garlic, crushed or grated
2 sprigs of rosemary, leaves removed and chopped
3 sprigs of thyme, leaves removed
165g (5¾oz) low-fat soft cheese
2 teaspoons salt
½ teaspoon black pepper
1.22kg (2lb 6oz) potatoes, cut into chips
170g (6oz) reduced fat Cheddar cheese, grated

Preheat the oven to 180°C fan/400°F/gas mark 6.

Place a large frying pan over a medium-high heat and add the butter. Once the butter is melted, add the leeks and cook for 7–8 minutes, stirring occasionally.

Meanwhile, mix together the garlic, rosemary, thyme, soft cheese, salt and pepper and set aside.

Add the potatoes to the pan and stir until well mixed with the leeks.

Pour the cheesy mixture over the top and bring to a simmer.

Transfer everything into an ovenproof dish, sprinkle over the Cheddar and bake in the oven for 40–50 minutes.

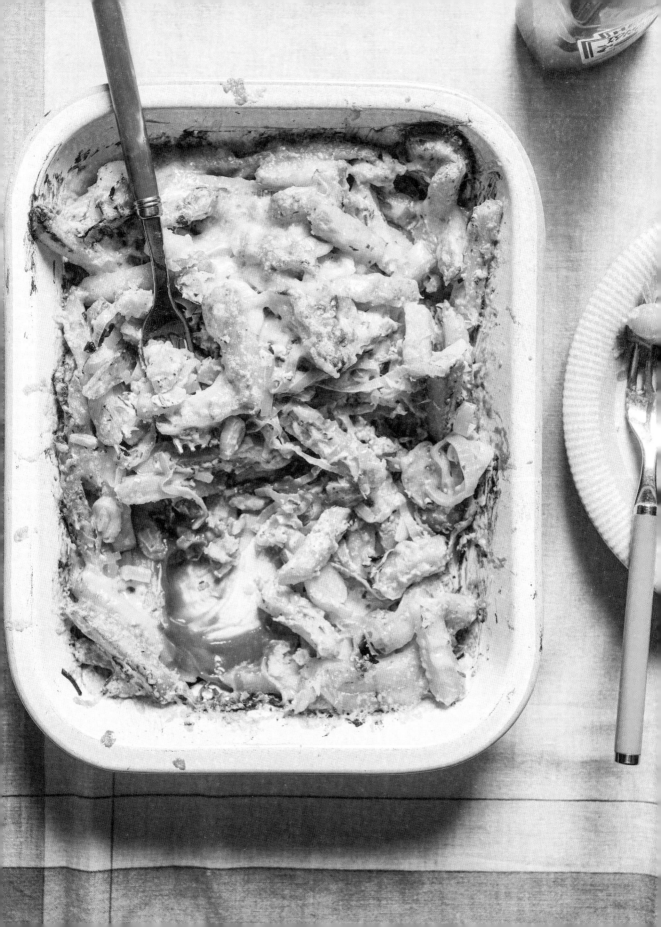

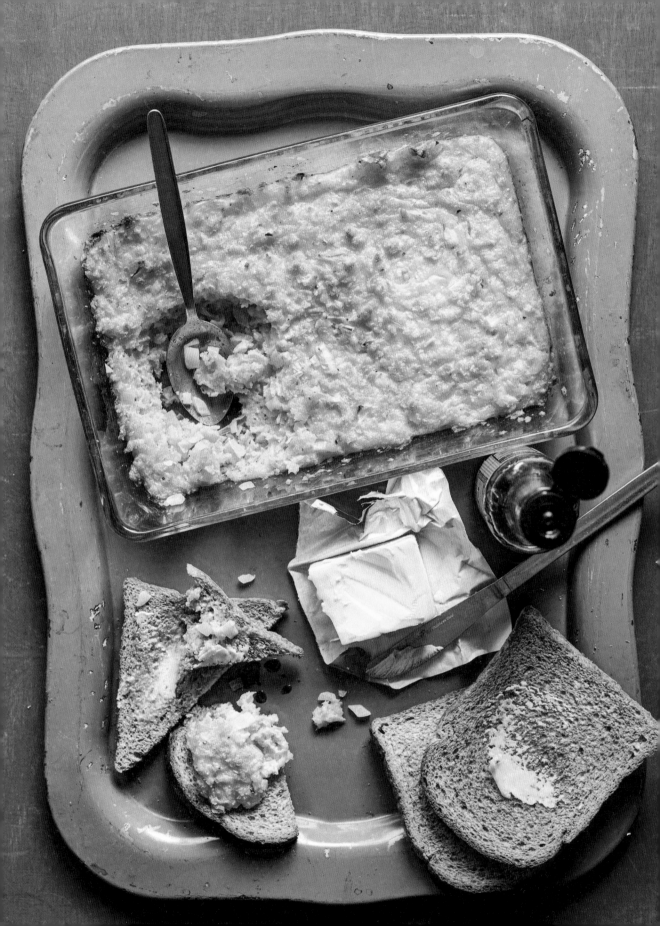

DOROTHY'S CHEESE PUD ON TOAST

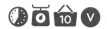

This is very much one of those recipes that looks like nothing at all but perfectly sums up an easy evening meal dish. It comes from memories of my nana (which sounds like a Yankee Candle scent, doesn't it), who would have this atop thickly buttered toast and nothing else. I haven't gussied up the recipe too much save to add some panko breadcrumbs, which I think helps to bring it all together, but you can leave it out if you wish.

Of course, for the full Dorothy experience, you should also use the absolute cheapest cheese you can find, then double the onion and halve the cheese to save a few extra pence on your shopping bill, then eat it off a padded tray you bought at Presto while your television blares loud enough to make blood pool in your eardrums. I've said it before: I do miss her.

SERVES: 4
PREP: 5 minutes
COOK: 30 minutes
CALORIES: 419

3 large eggs
200g (7oz) reduced-fat extra
   mature Cheddar cheese, grated
25g (1oz) panko breadcrumbs
1 large onion, finely diced
a pinch of salt and black pepper
wholemeal bread, toasted

Preheat the oven to 170°C fan/375°F/gas mark 5.

Spray an ovenproof dish with a little oil. Mix all the ingredients except the bread together in a bowl and tip into the dish.

Bake in the oven for 30 minutes. It's cooked when it still has a bit of a wobble, but then you spoon it out and slap it on some toast – lovely.

NOTES

As Paul and I are a little frou-frou, we sometimes have this as a thick 'omelette' on top of a bagel with bacon, but that's getting ahead of ourselves.

Some wholegrain mustard would work a treat here.

GOAT'S CHEESE CHEESECAKES

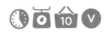

We have some cheek including these as a dinner idea, but listen, sometimes you just need something light for your evening meal, and these are just the ticket. If you can't be bothered faffing about with caramelising your onions, then by all means use the jarred stuff from the supermarket. That's the thing with evening meals: sometimes you want to spend the evening making conversation over the oven, other times you want something quick and tasty with minimal fuss.

And anyway! This is our book, and we bloody love cheesecake, and in the absence of being able to put an actual cheesecake in there, this is the next best thing. We serve these with a side salad of simple dressed leaves that always looks super left on the plate for the dog to take care of afterwards. Honestly, that's the best thing about Goomba – saves us any amount of money on dishwasher tablets.

MAKES: 4
PREP: 5 minutes
COOK: 25 minutes
CALORIES: 285

2 red onions, finely sliced
1 teaspoon fresh thyme leaves
1 tablespoon soft brown sugar
4 tablespoons balsamic vinegar
4 oatcakes
150g (5½oz) soft goat's cheese
150g (5½oz) reduced-fat cream
    cheese

Spray a frying pan with a little oil and place over a medium-low heat. Add the sliced onions and thyme and cook for 15–20 minutes, stirring occasionally, until soft and golden.

Add the sugar, balsamic vinegar and 2 tablespoons of water and cook for another 5 minutes. Set aside to cool.

Meanwhile, put the oatcakes into a sandwich bag and bash with a rolling pin until they resemble breadcrumbs.

Divide the oatcake crumbs between four individual ramekins (or use one big one).

Mix together the goat's cheese and cream cheese in a bowl and gently spoon into the ramekins on top of the oatcake crumbs.

Top with the caramelised onions.

NOTES

Those little Gü glass ramekins you've been saving for years are perfect for this!

Serve as is for a tasty lunch or brunch, or with a salad for a top dinner.

You can swap the fresh thyme for ¼ teaspoon of dried if you prefer.

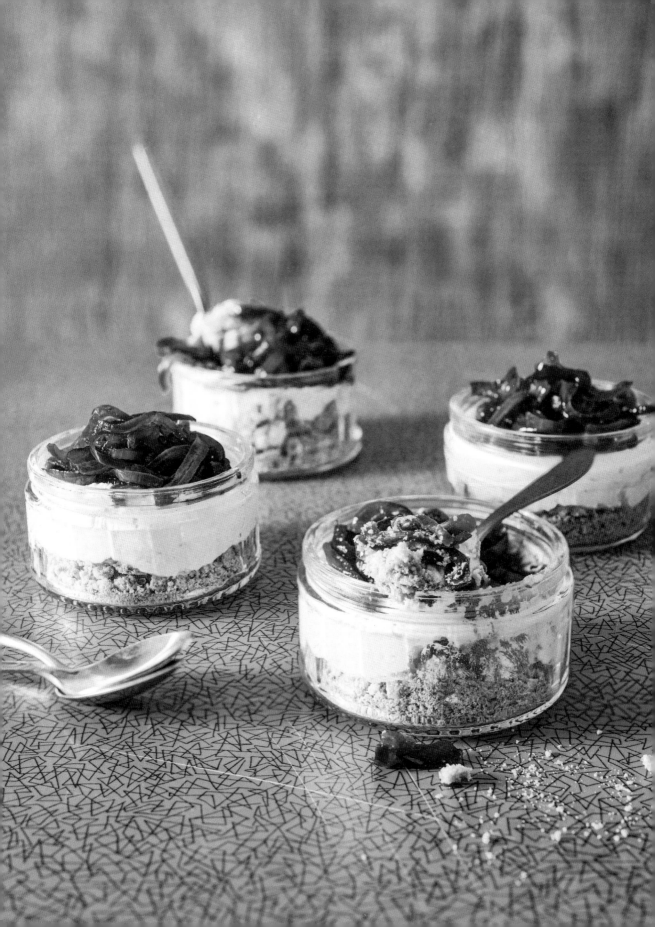

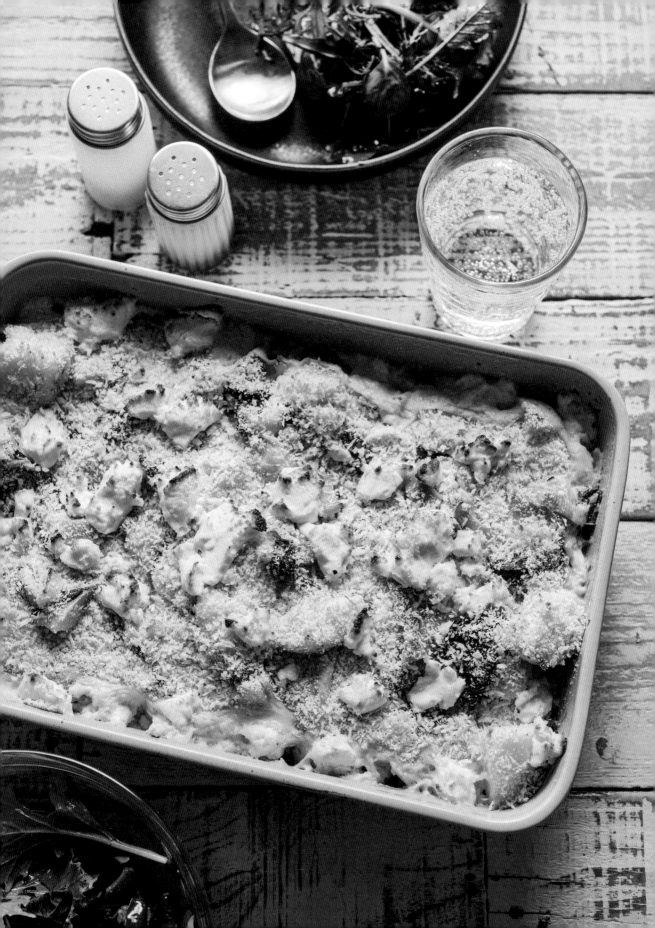

EASY CHEESY GRATIN

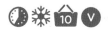

This cheesy, bubbling, burbling meal is a delight and you must try it without delay, for nourishment will be your reward. You could gussy it up with the addition of bacon and/or sausages if you want, but we encourage you to let the dish stand on its own two feet.

Meanwhile, speaking of cheese, I wanted to update on the previous two book entries about health anxiety. It may come across as indulgent to throw this into a recipe intro, but nevertheless: everything is going well. I'm rarely troubled with the anxiety that used to be all-encompassing and crippling, and that's despite all the health excitement in the news. I only mention it here because if you're out there and you're struggling and you think it will never get better, take it from a fat lad who loves to gab that it absolutely will. You've got this!

SERVES: 4
PREP: 10 minutes
COOK: 45 minutes
CALORIES: 488

900g (2lb) potatoes, cut into 2cm chunks
4 leeks, sliced thinly
300ml (10fl oz) vegetable stock
200g (7oz) baby spinach
200g (7oz) low-fat soft cheese
100g (3½oz) fat-free cottage cheese
50g (1¾oz) panko breadcrumbs
200g (7oz) soft goat's cheese

Preheat the oven to 220°C fan/475°F/gas mark 9.

Bring a large pan of salted water to the boil and add the potatoes. Cook for 15–20 minutes until tender, then drain and keep to one side.

Meanwhile, spray a large saucepan with a little oil and place over a medium heat. Add the leeks and cook for 4–5 minutes, stirring occasionally.

Add the stock, stir, then reduce the heat to low and simmer for 8 minutes.

Add the spinach to the pan a handful at a time and cook until wilted.

Add the drained potatoes to the pan along with the soft cheese and cottage cheese, stir, bring to a simmer, then remove from the heat.

Pour the mixture into an ovenproof dish and sprinkle over the panko breadcrumbs. Crumble the goat's cheese over the top and bake in the oven for 10 minutes until lightly browned and crispy.

NOTE

We never peel our potatoes, but feel free to do so if you prefer!

FRENCH ONION QUICHE

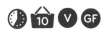

You know who has no time for quiche? DCI Kenneth Sexington. He's a bloke who will only accept a lunch if he can feel his arteries harden as he swallows. He's the type of no-nonsense guy who will throw the cheese & onion crisps out of the multipack because they don't make his eyes water the same way that salt & vinegar do. He hasn't had a feeling since his wife left him in 1989 for the leader of the local darts team, and he's just fine with that. Her loss. The 'H' on his bathroom taps shines as new as the first day he had the bathroom put in: he enjoys a shower as cold as the love for his daughter and dries himself with the printed profiles of all the scum he's put away over the years. He has no time for quiche. He has no time for criminals. But most of all: DCI Kenneth Sexington has no time for *you*.

Well, he had to make an appearance at some point. To most of you, that whole paragraph will mean absolutely nothing. But to those that know, it's always good to catch up with an old friend. The quiche recipe below is absolutely killer (because of course it is) and you must simply trust us with the potato. We promise it's good.

SERVES: 4
PREP: 15 minutes
COOK: 1 hour 15 minutes
CALORIES: 340

1 large sweet potato, peeled
3 large onions
45g (1¾oz) butter
100g (3½oz) reduced-fat crème fraîche
2 large egg yolks
100ml (3½fl oz) milk
2 large eggs
40g (1½oz) Gruyère cheese
salt and black pepper

NOTE

Gruyère is the traditional cheese used for anything French onion, but any cheese will do.

Preheat the oven to 190°C fan/410°F/gas mark 7.

Slice the sweet potato into thick rounds, about ½cm (¼ inch) thick. Spray a flan dish with a little oil and lay the potato slices in the bottom, overlapping, and a little bit up the sides. It doesn't need to be too neat! This will make your quiche base. Give it another spray of oil.

Bake in the oven for 25 minutes, then remove from the oven and set aside.

While the sweet potatoes are cooking, peel, halve and thinly slice the onions. Place a frying pan over a medium-low heat, add the butter, and stir until melted. Add the onions and a generous pinch of salt, and cook for 30 minutes, stirring occasionally. Increase the heat to medium and cook for another 15 minutes, until just starting to crisp (reduce the heat if they're cooking too quickly).

Meanwhile, mix the crème fraîche with the 2 egg yolks and whisk until smooth. Gradually add the milk and the 2 whole eggs, mix in the Gruyère, and season with a bit of salt and pepper.

Spread three-quarters of the onions over the potato base, then pour over the egg mix. Sprinkle the rest of the onions on top and bake in the oven for 30 minutes, until nicely wobbly (cook for a few extra minutes if it hasn't yet cooked through enough).

Remove from the oven and allow to cool enough to remove from the dish.

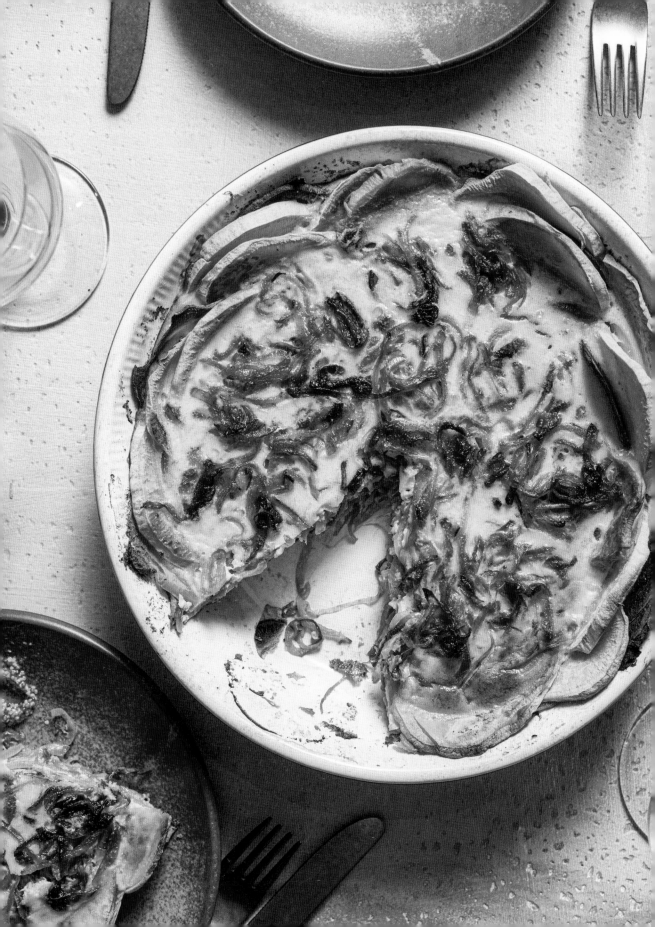

AUBERGINE PARMO

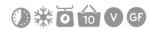

Perhaps you're thinking 'James and Paul, you put a recipe in the last book for a parmo, and I am aghast you've had the audacity to slip another one in.' Perhaps you're right. But let us beg mercy for a moment: it was one of the most popular recipes we have ever done, and we wanted to make a true vegetarian alternative that wasn't just 'replace the chicken with Quorn', as some others may have done. This is a fresher and lighter take and we implore you to give it a go, even if you're a confirmed carnivore who brushes their teeth with a rasher of freshly cooked bacon.

If you wanted to be decadent – and understand we encourage decadence in all things – you could melt some herby soft cheese down and slosh it around the recipe as you layer it up. Admittedly, it then tips the whole dish more towards a rustic (for rustic, read slapdash) moussaka, but if you don't tell the police then nor shall we.

SERVES: 4
PREP: 10 minutes
COOK: 1 hour
CALORIES: 293

2 large aubergines, sliced
1 × 400g (14oz) tin of chopped tomatoes
500ml (18fl oz) passata
½ teaspoon black pepper
1 teaspoon dried mixed herbs
1 × 400g (14oz) tin of butter beans
1 mozzarella ball, torn into small pieces
50g (1¾oz) panko breadcrumbs (optional)
a bunch of fresh basil, leaves picked

Preheat the oven to 180°C fan/400°F/gas mark 6.

Spray a large frying pan with a little oil and place it over a medium-high heat. Add the sliced aubergines to the pan in batches, and cook for 8–10 minutes each side, until nicely browned.

Mix together the chopped tomatoes, passata, black pepper and mixed herbs, and pour one third of the mixture into the bottom of a large casserole dish.

Spread half the butter beans over the tomatoes and top with slices of aubergine and a third of the mozzarella.

Repeat with another layer of tomatoes, the rest of the beans, aubergine and cheese, and finish with a final layer of tomatoes and mozzarella. If using panko breadcrumbs, sprinkle evenly over the top.

Bake in the oven for 35–40 minutes.

Sprinkle over the chopped basil and serve.

NOTE

If freezing, freeze before baking. Defrost thoroughly before baking.

If gluten-free, find alternative to panko breadcrumbs (if using).

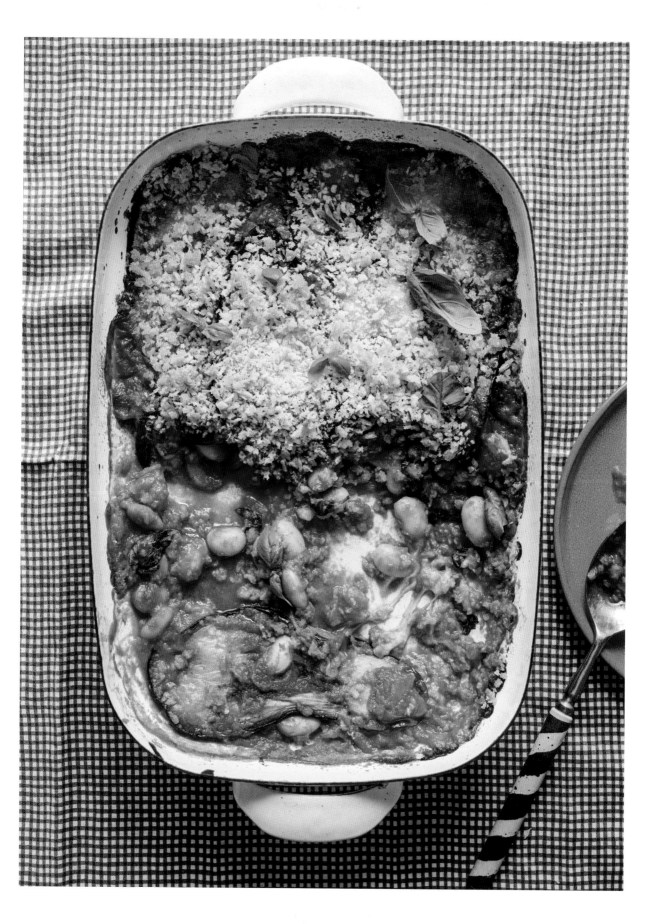

ANGLESEY EGGS

Anglesey eggs is one of our go-to dishes when we have leftover mash, as you can save a lot of time here if you don't need to fart about with the potatoes. Of course, the concept of leftovers in our house is as alien as monogamy or putting a new bin-liner in the bin after you've emptied it, but you catch our drift. This cheesy, starchy bowl of deliciousness needs to get to the top of your 'give it a try' list.

As Paul mentions in the notes, you're not beholden to Caerphilly cheese – in fact, I rather suspect he only uses it because he knows how I'll agonise over how to spell it and whether to capitalise it. To our Welsh friends, if we have it wrong, then *Mae'n ddrwg gen i*.

Gosh, I do hope Google Translate hasn't had a fit and said something awful right there.

SERVES: 4
PREP: 10 minutes
COOK: 50 minutes
CALORIES: 497

4 eggs
1 large leek, sliced
750g (1lb 10oz) potatoes
30g (1oz) butter
2 tablespoons low-fat soft cheese
500ml (18fl oz) milk
30g (1oz) plain flour
100g (3½oz) Caerphilly cheese, crumbled
40g (1½oz) panko breadcrumbs

Preheat the oven to 200°C fan/425°F/gas mark 7.

Bring a pan of water to the boil and cook the eggs for 8 minutes, then drain, peel under cold running water, quarter and set aside.

Spray a saucepan with a little oil and place over a medium heat. Add the leeks and cook for 5 minutes, until softened.

Meanwhile, bring a large pan of salted water to the boil. Chop the potatoes into 2cm (¾ inch) cubes (no need to peel) and add to the boiling water for 10 minutes.

Drain the potatoes, then put back into the pan along with half the butter, the soft cheese and a splash of milk (if needed), and mash until smooth.

Add the leeks to the potatoes and mix well.

Spray a large ovenproof dish with a little oil and spoon the mash into it. Lay the eggs on top of the mash.

Place the leek pan back over a medium heat. Add the remaining butter, the flour and the milk and whisk continuously until smooth, then simmer for 2 minutes.

Add half the Caerphilly cheese and cook for another 2 minutes.

Pour the sauce over the mash and eggs, and sprinkle over the remaining cheese and the panko breadcrumbs. Bake in the oven for 15–20 minutes.

NOTES

Wensleydale, Cheshire and Cheddar could be used instead, if you don't fancy Caerphilly.

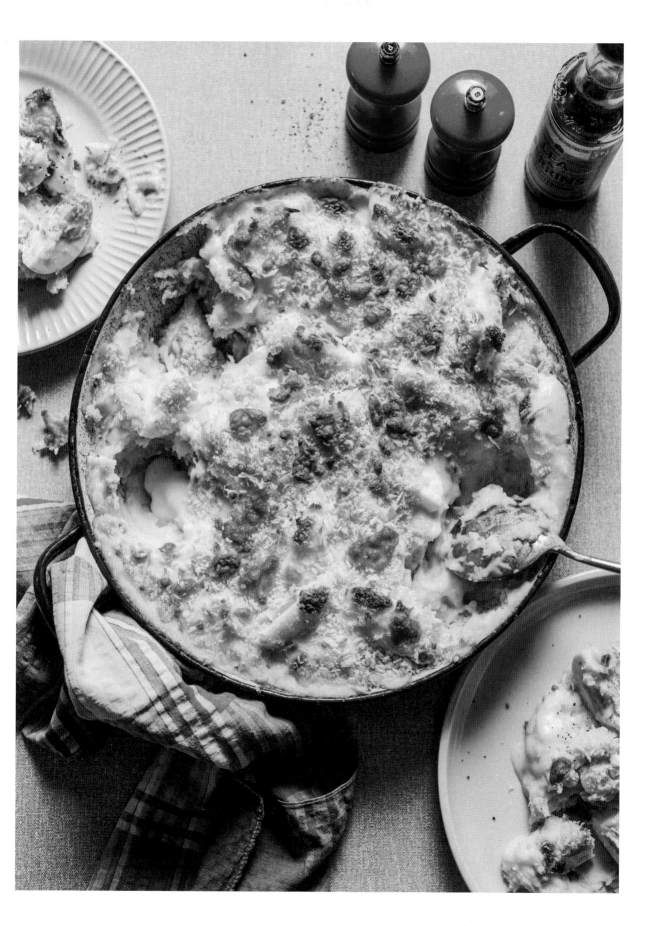

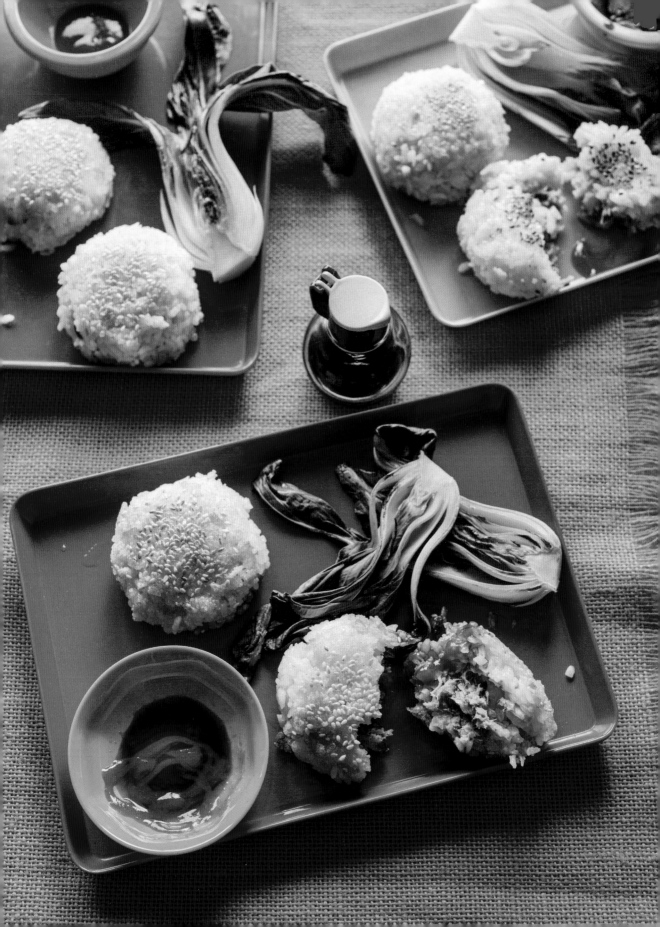

SPICY JAPANESE RICE BALLS

Sticky Japanese balls are presented here for your kind attention. Similarly, Paul and I were lucky to take a trip to Tokyo a couple of years ago, before COVID ruined everything, and boy, did we manage a fair few Japanese sticky balls on that trip.

But what a place! I do sometimes wish we were the sort of couple who visit new countries and stand agog at the culture and wonders, but no. Generally speaking, our holidays consist of us going to the most outlandish places to eat, hurling ourselves off something high, sampling the locals, and taking photos with pretend sad faces. Tokyo was no exception: within a couple of hours we had enjoyed dinner in a hedgehog café and won a plushie the size of Paul from a giant crane machine.

The absolute pinnacle of that trip was us both turning up to a very fancy restaurant with neither of us a) liking fish, or b) realising it was an exclusively seafood place. We aren't ones for being impolite, so we pretended each last morsel was delicious, and spent every moment when our hosts' backs were turned tipping the meal into our rucksacks. It was a very pricy affair, but we had fun, and it's not like I ever need an excuse to buy a new bag.

SERVES: 4
PREP: 25 minutes
COOK: 15 minutes
CALORIES: 281

300g (10½oz) sushi rice
¼ teaspoon salt
1 × 145g tin of tuna chunks, drained
2 tablespoons reduced-fat mayonnaise
1 tablespoon rice vinegar
½ teaspoon lemon juice
2 teaspoons sriracha
1 gherkin, grated
1 shallot, grated
2 cloves of garlic, crushed
¼ teaspoon chilli flakes
1 teaspoon sesame seeds

Place the rice in a bowl and add just enough water to cover. Gently rub the rice between your fingers until the water is cloudy, then drain and repeat a couple more times until the water is clear. Place the rice in a saucepan and add 600ml (20fl oz) of water and the salt. Bring to the boil, then cover with a lid, reduce the heat to low and cook for 10 minutes. Drain and leave to cool.

Meanwhile, in a bowl mix together the tuna, mayonnaise, rice vinegar, lemon juice, sriracha, gherkin, shallot, garlic and chilli flakes, then set aside.

Once the rice has cooled, divide it into 8 rough-shaped portions. With wet hands, spread the rice out into a burger shape in your hand and spoon in 1–2 tablespoons of the tuna mix, then gently fold the rice over it to make a ball-like shape. Gently flatten it into a puck shape, then repeat with the rest of the rice and filling (washing your hands in between makes this easier). Sprinkle over the sesame seeds.

Place a large frying pan over a medium-high heat and spray with a little oil. Add the rice balls and cook for 2–3 minutes each side, until browned and crispy.

Serve!

NOTE

These are lovely with steamed greens, and make a great alternative to the usual rice with curry.

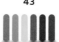

PRAWN SAGANAKI

Our quest to find a home for the prawn other than 'bought with good intentions and binned with lament' continues at quite the pace, with this saganaki dish proving tasty enough to circumvent my irrational fear of prawns. It's those little spindly bits that freak me out: I always imagine them lightly touching my lips or brushing against my moustache hair and it feeling utterly terrifying. Paul doesn't share this fear, but how could he? He set about growing a beard back in 2013 and has only just now reached the point where his chin-ripples are covered.

But then my life is full of irrationalities – I don't like deep kitchen drawers because I'm always convinced I'll slip my hand into the darkness and impale myself on an apple corer. Similarly, I don't like parking anywhere near a drain because I just know I'm one impulsive moment away from posting my phone smartly into the sewers. Paul doesn't like blowing up balloons – not because he's scared of the pop but rather of laughing and somehow ingesting the deflated balloon into his windpipe.

And we shouldn't get started on crumpets and sponges, because that is a hellscape I shall never return from. Where were we? Ah yes, the prawn. Terrifying, but so tasty.

SERVES: 4
PREP: 10 minutes
COOK: 30 minutes
CALORIES: 166

250g (9oz) king prawns, peeled
1 onion, finely diced
3 cloves of garlic, crushed
   or grated
1 green pepper, finely diced
1 teaspoon tomato purée
½ teaspoon dried chilli flakes
1 × 400g (14oz) tin of chopped
   tomatoes
½ teaspoon sugar
1 large bunch of fresh basil,
   chopped
150g (5½oz) reduced-fat feta
   cheese
½ teaspoon dried oregano
salt and black pepper

Preheat the oven to 200°C fan/425°F/gas mark 7.

Spray a large pan with a little oil and place over a high heat. Add the prawns and a pinch of salt and pepper. Cook for 1 minute, until golden all over, then remove to a plate and set aside.

Reduce the heat to medium. Spray the pan with a bit more oil and add the onions. Cook for 1–2 minutes, then add the garlic, green pepper, tomato purée and dried chilli flakes and stir well for 1–2 minutes.

Add the tomatoes and sugar, stir, and bring to the boil. Add half the chopped basil and crumble in half the feta.

Gently put the prawns back into the pan and give a gentle stir. Crumble the rest of the feta on top, scatter over the basil and sprinkle over the dried oregano.

Transfer to the oven and bake for 20 minutes, then serve.

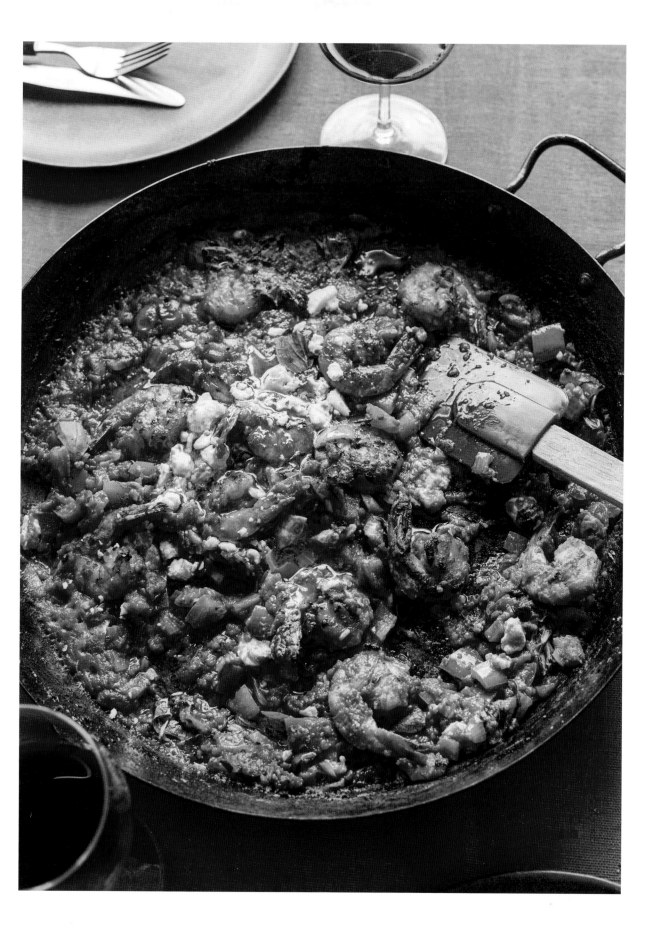

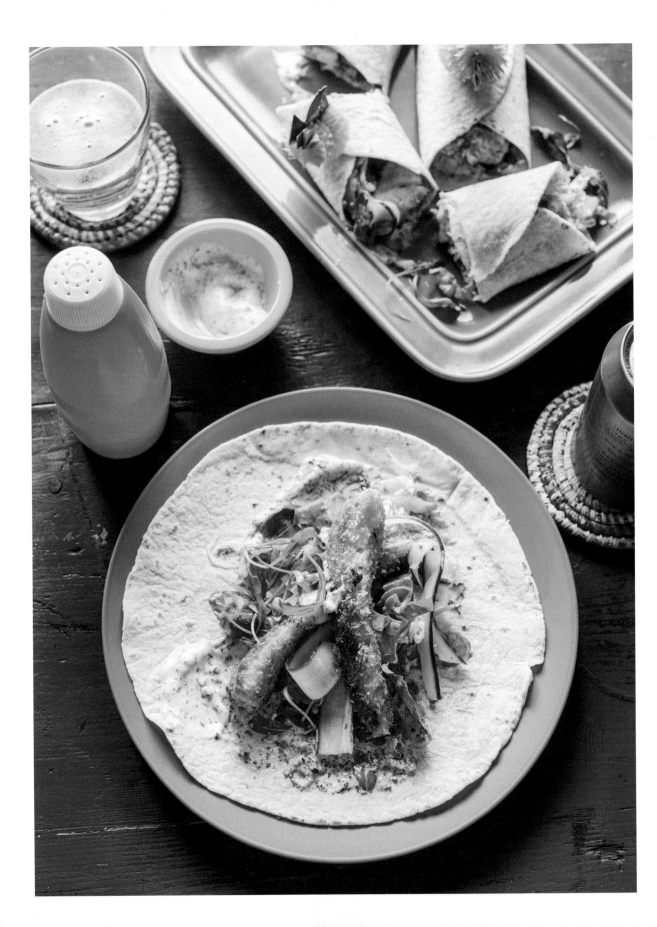

BATTERED HADDOCK WRAPS

One of two recipes inspired by my North Coast 500 trip comes via what was simply the best street-food meal I had on that trip, courtesy of the Seafood Shack in Ullapool. Towards the end of my trip, with a slight hankering for home and the jiggliness of Paul's comforting bosom, I found myself mincing around Ullapool with no plan other than to see where I ended up. I walked past the Seafood Shack a couple of times, forever perturbed by the thought of seafood, but it smelled so wonderfully inviting that somehow, just somehow, my fat cankles steered me in.

I'm so glad they did: I had a battered fish wrap and it was utterly divine. I don't want to get evangelical here, but I've never had seafood done so well, either before or since. It was the first thing I told Paul about after I got home, once we'd discussed at length the charges to our American Express card and the fact all of my jeans had grass-stains on the knees. While we will not pretend that this matches their wrap, it is a good alternative for those on a lower-calorie kick.

If you're up in Ullapool, do give them a visit. Otherwise, please bask in the glory that is this wonder.

SERVES: 4
PREP: 15 minutes
COOK: 12 minutes
CALORIES: 318

50g (1¾oz) panko breadcrumbs
zest of 1 lemon
4 tablespoons tartare sauce
1 tablespoon dried parsley
1 egg, beaten
400g (14oz) haddock, cut into
    8–10 fingers
4 tortilla wraps
½ cucumber, deseeded and
    cut into strips
25g (1oz) rocket
1 little gem lettuce, finely sliced

Mix together the panko breadcrumbs and lemon zest.

Mix the tartare sauce with the parsley and set aside.

Lay out two shallow dishes, one with the beaten egg and another with the panko breadcrumbs.

Spray a large frying pan with a little oil and place over a medium heat.

Gently dip the fish into the beaten egg, then coat with the panko breadcrumbs. Place the fish in the pan and cook for 4–5 minutes each side.

Spread some tartare sauce over each tortilla and top with the cucumber, rocket and lettuce.

Add the cooked fish fingers, wrap and enjoy.

WOR PAUL'S BAGGED PLAICE

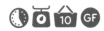

We have to make a confession here: this recipe is very commonly known as fish en papillote, which translates as fish cooked in parchment (I think, anyway: I studied Spanish at school, as our French teacher's moustache used to terrify me to the point I couldn't concentrate in the lesson). You may have seen similar recipes, as it is a common way of cooking fish to make sure it doesn't dry out. However, we're calling it 'Wor Paul's Bagged Plaice' because we really, really wanted a *RuPaul's Drag Race* pun in this book.

Utterly shameless, we know.

We would both absolutely love to be given a drag makeover – it's very high up on the list of things to do before we're forty, just below divorce. Neither of us could attempt it ourselves and give the process the respect it deserves: I have a job just managing to brush my teeth without setting fire to my face, let alone applying make-up, so best leave it to the experts. A dear friend of mine, Astrid Zeneca (always wonderfully fabulous), has offered to do us both, but I'm not convinced even she has enough Ronseal and caulk in her bag of tricks to make us look stunning.

Still, given the way Ru works, there'll probably be a *Drag Race* series based on the residents of our street soon, so …

SERVES: 4
PREP: 10 minutes
COOK: 20 minutes
CALORIES: 180

3 tablespoons fresh parsley, finely chopped
2 cloves of garlic, crushed or grated
zest and juice of 1 lemon
4 small handfuls of baby spinach
4 fish portions (about 500–650g/ 1lb 2oz–1lb 7oz) – we've used plaice (mainly for the pun in the title, to be honest), but any white fish will do
4 spring onions, sliced
2 tablespoons butter
salt and black pepper

Preheat the oven to 230°C fan/475°F/gas mark 9.

Mix together the parsley, garlic and lemon zest in a small bowl, and set aside.

Tear off 4 large squares of greaseproof paper. Place a handful of spinach in the centre of each square (1 square per person) and place the fish on top, then sprinkle over the lemon juice and spring onions, and spoon on the butter. Add a pinch of salt and pepper, and top with the parsley mix.

Bring the edges of the paper together, then scrunch and gently twist to seal.

Bake in the oven for 10 minutes until the fish is opaque throughout and flakey.

NOTE

Cod, bass, pollock and salmon all work really well!

Serve with one of our veg 5 ways (pages 160–161) for a tasty dinner.

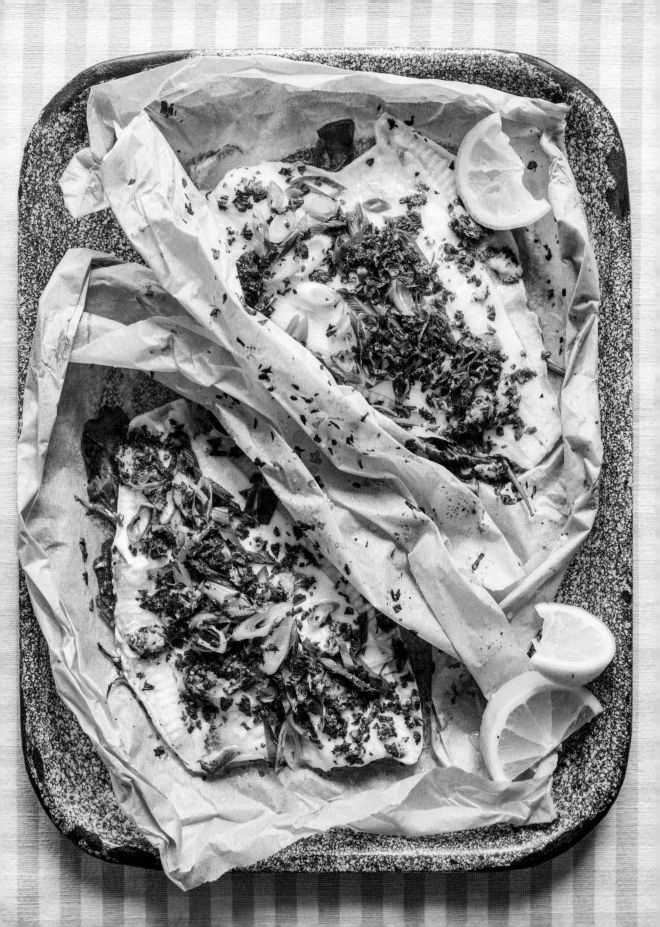

KEDGEREE

There are so many ways of doing kedgeree that any attempt at a definitive recipe will fall on its a*se, so this is our take on a fishy dinner. This did take a lot of getting my head around, and indeed, it was only because kedgeree appeared in a meal-delivery service we were trialling that we even gave it the light of day. But, possibly because it isn't too fishy and there are a lot of complementary flavours in this pan, it's absolutely worth a gamble!

SERVES: 4
PREP: 10 minutes
COOK: 50 minutes
CALORIES: 364

200g (7oz) boneless haddock fillets
1 onion, finely diced
1 green chilli, finely diced
2cm (¾ inch) piece of root ginger, grated
1 tablespoon curry powder
½ teaspoon garam masala
½ teaspoon ground cumin
¼ teaspoon ground turmeric
1 teaspoon mustard seeds
200g (7oz) basmati rice
600ml (20fl oz) vegetable stock
150g (5½oz) frozen peas
2 large eggs
4 tablespoons fat-free natural yoghurt
1 bunch of chives, chopped
½ lemon

Preheat the oven to 180°C fan/400°F/gas mark 6.

Place the haddock on a sheet of tin foil and spray with a little oil, then wrap in the foil. Bake in the oven for 15 minutes, until the fish is opaque and flakes easily.

Meanwhile, spray a large frying pan with a little oil and place over a medium heat. Add the onion and green chilli and cook for 5–6 minutes, until the onion is starting to turn golden.

Add the ginger, curry powder, garam masala, cumin, turmeric and mustard seeds and cook for another 2 minutes.

Add the rice and give a good stir, then pour in the vegetable stock and the frozen peas, stirring once more. Bring everything to a simmer, then reduce the heat to low, cover with a lid and cook for 15 minutes.

Remove the haddock from the oven and break up with a fork. Add to the frying pan and stir gently to combine.

Bring a small saucepan of water to the boil and boil the eggs for 7 minutes, then rinse under cold water, peel and cut into quarters.

Serve the kedgeree on plates and top with the eggs, yoghurt, chives and a squeeze of lemon juice.

NOTE

Tinned mackerel is a great alternative to haddock here – simply heat and add to the frying pan.

If gluten-free, make sure your curry powder is free-from gluten.

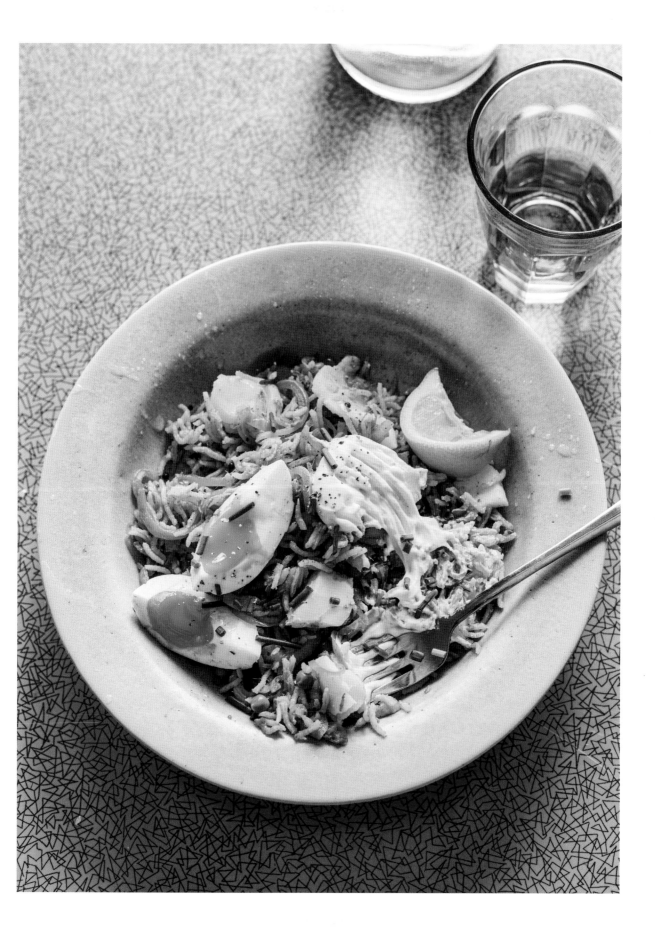

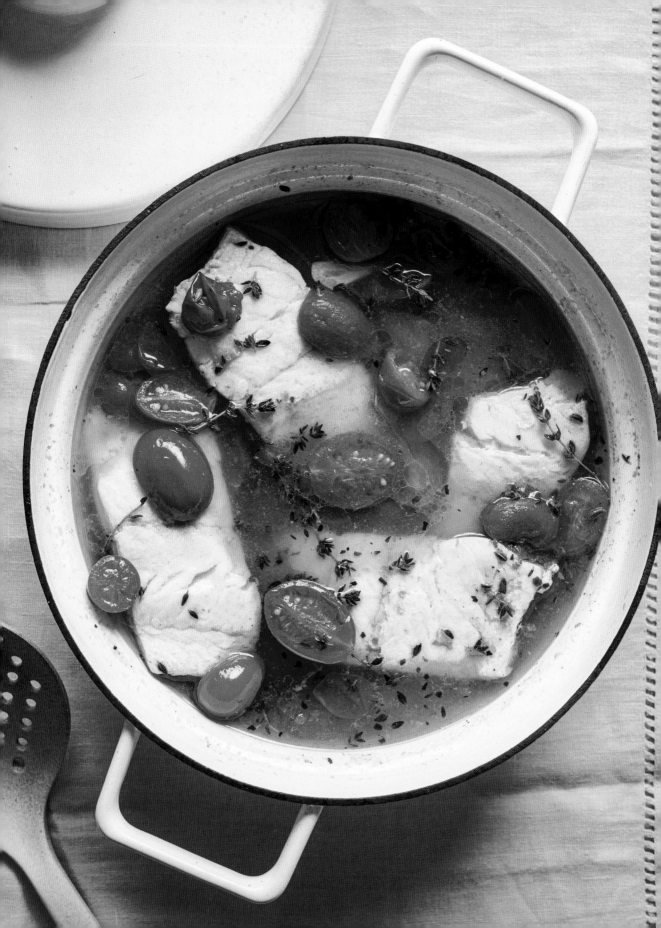

FISH IN CRAZY WATER

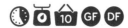

No really, that's what it's called. 'Pesce all'acqua pazza' is the 'official' name, and doesn't that sound far better tripping off the tongue? Well, it probably does in the mouth of some handsome Italian waiter who you know would treat you terribly but would give you a good night. I long for a romance that I can sell to *Take a Break* a few months later when it all goes wrong. Any excuse to put on some comfortable pyjamas, stare sadly into a lens and adopt a '*I fort 'e were diffrent*' face. Anyhoo.

Crazy water is a delightfully lyrical way of describing the spicy broth that the fish is poached in, but as recipes that may change the way you view fish go, this is a blinder. You can add all sorts here and when it comes to serving, some plain potatoes or some bread to soak up the broth is lovely.

Just a note on seasoning – as there are a lot of different flavours jostling for position in this pan, make sure you taste as you go. We add a pinch of salt, though it often isn't needed, but that's on you to check.

SERVES: 4
PREP: 5 minutes
COOK: 25 minutes
CALORIES: 203

2 cloves of garlic, thinly sliced
½ teaspoon fennel seeds
¼ teaspoon dried chilli flakes
400g (14oz) cherry tomatoes, halved
175ml (6fl oz) white wine
2 teaspoons dried oregano
2 teaspoons fresh thyme leaves
4 cod fillets

Spray a frying pan with a little oil and place over a medium-low heat. Add the garlic and fennel seeds and cook for 1–2 minutes, until the garlic starts to sizzle. Add the chilli flakes and cook for 1 more minute, stirring frequently.

Add the tomatoes and cook for 2–3 minutes, stirring gently now and again. Add the wine, oregano, thyme and a pinch of salt, along with 500ml (18fl oz) of water. Cover the pan and simmer for 10 minutes, then remove the lid and cook for a further 2 minutes.

Gently place the fish in the pan, cover again, and cook for 5–7 minutes until opaque and flakey.

Serve.

NOTE

We used cod, but any white fish will do. Haddock, pollock, hake, sea bream and sea bass are good alternatives.

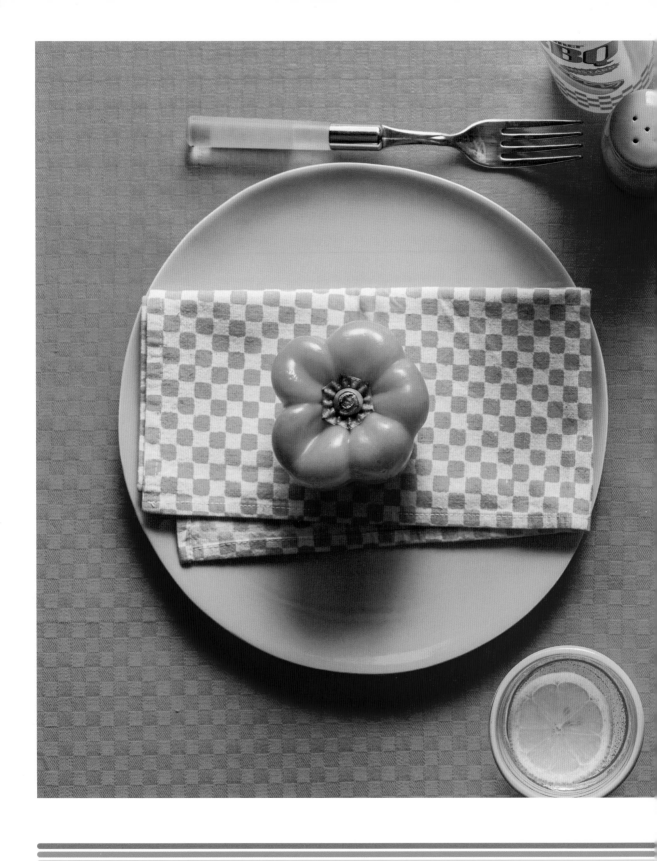

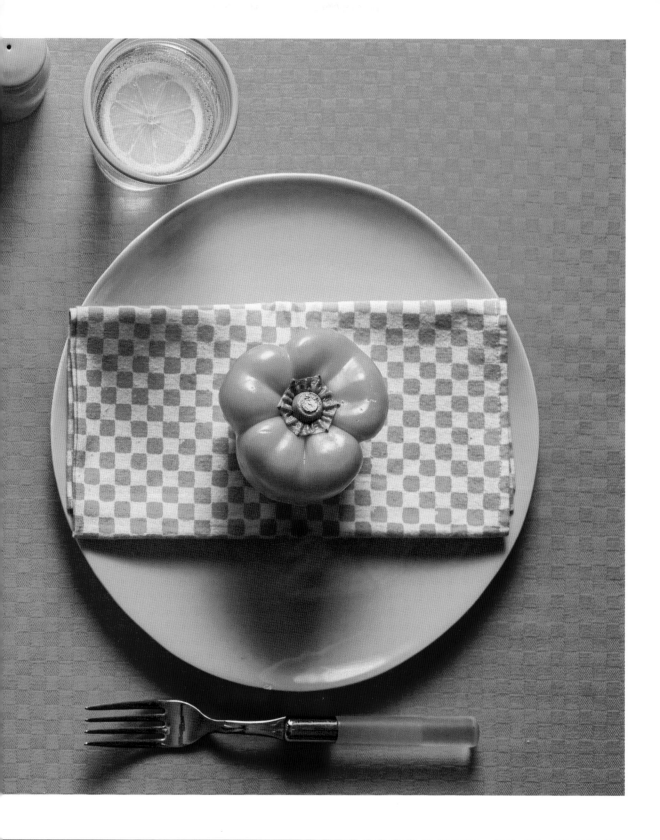

PASTA

THAT FAMOUS FETA PASTA RECIPE
(YOU KNOW THE ONE)

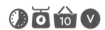

We have included this recipe because good lord, it was absolutely everywhere for a good month or two and, after spending too much time thinking we were above TikTok trends, we finally caved in and gave it a go. Absolutely worth all the hullabaloo. Now, we have kept it simple here, but we have made versions of this with quartered red onions, which works a treat, and also those tiny pickled onions you can sometimes find in the fancy aisle in Tesco. Yours to explore.

We can't get away with TikTok, though: we're simply far too old, and in the way, to do it with any conviction. That said, if you will indulge us for a moment, we do have a recommendation. Our good friend Adam has carved himself a little niche on TikTok doing all sorts of wholesome content, including biscuit reviews and showing off his incredibly bald head. With the fervent hope that he hasn't started posting problematic content in the short time between us writing this and the book going to print, we encourage you to take a look at @Adcro. Tell him we sent you.

SERVES: 4
PREP: 5 minutes
COOK: 40 minutes
CALORIES: 479

200g (7oz) reduced-fat feta
475g (1lb) cherry tomatoes
3 long sweet red peppers, sliced into … well, slices
¼ teaspoon dried chilli flakes
400g (14oz) penne
4 cloves of garlic, finely chopped
a handful of fresh basil leaves
salt and black pepper

Preheat the oven to 200°C fan/425°F/gas mark 7.

Place the block of feta in the middle of a baking dish and surround with the cherry tomatoes and peppers. Spray with a little oil, and sprinkle over the chilli flakes.

Bake in the oven for 30 minutes, then increase the temperature to 230°C fan/475°F/gas mark 9 and cook for another 5–10 minutes, until the tomatoes and feta have browned.

Meanwhile, bring a large pan of salted water to the boil. Add the pasta and cook according to the packet instructions, then drain (remembering to reserve half a mugful of water for later).

When the tomatoes and feta have finished cooking, remove from the oven, add the garlic and basil, and give a quick, gentle stir. Add the drained pasta and continue to stir gently until everything is well combined, adding a splash of pasta water if needed.

Season with salt and pepper and serve!

NOTE

We used penne for this but really, any pasta is absolutely fine.

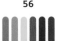

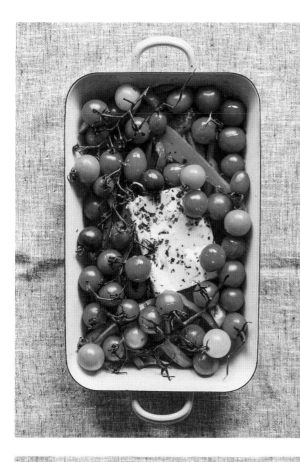
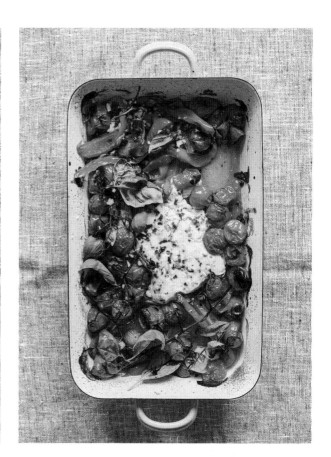
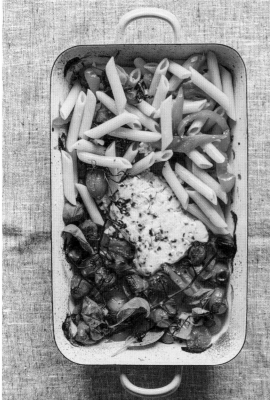
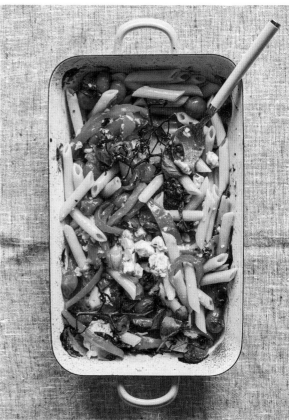

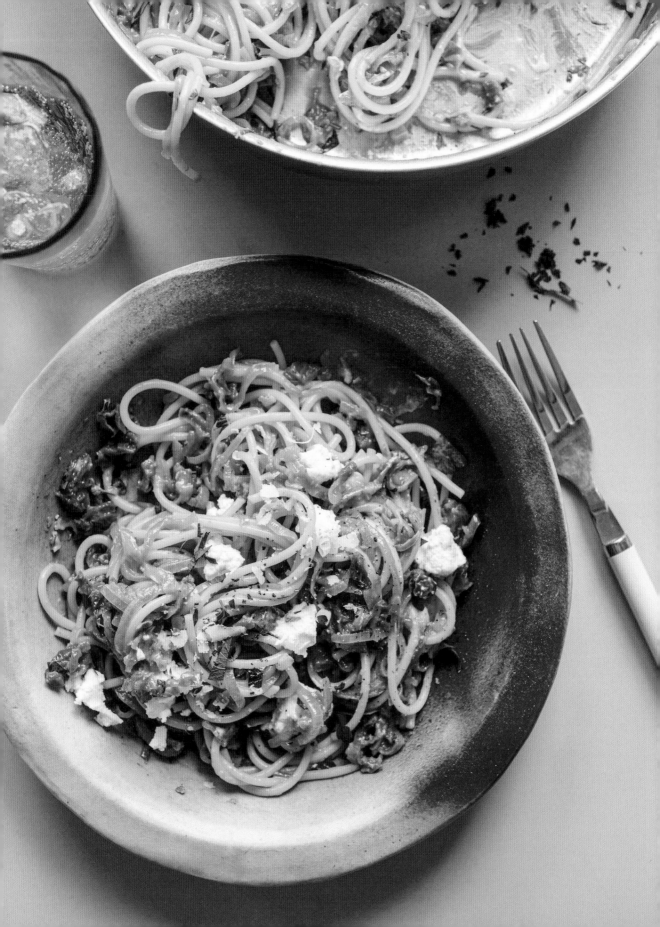

CARAMELISED ONION PASTA

You know the drill by now when it comes to our pasta dishes. They're never extravagant, they're never fussy and you almost certainly wouldn't write home about them. But then again, why would you write home about anything? The only time I think I would ever write home to Paul is to tell him I'd met another man and was eloping to Scarborough to run an antiques shop and spend my evenings laughing gaily over an elegant supper. And even then, he would never see the letter because he would do what he always does with post, whether it's junk mail, a blackmail letter or a court summons, and that's stick it on top of the bookcase because *somehow* that's easier than shredding it. We live our matrimonial life on a knife-edge.

But back to the pasta (and I *do* feel better for that, thank you) – this is one of those dishes you can lazily cobble together on an evening when your feet hurt and your life is fuzzy with stress, and it will, I guarantee, bring you all levels of joy. Plus there's wine in it, which means that when you're finished adding it to the dish, you can drink the rest with the other bottle you bought on the way home. Let's not pretend.

SERVES: 4
PREP: 10 minutes
COOK: 45 minutes
CALORIES: 496

1 tablespoon rapeseed oil
3 onions, finely sliced
4 cloves of garlic, crushed
   or grated
1 tablespoon balsamic vinegar
300g (10½oz) spaghetti
1 teaspoon dried mixed herbs
70ml (2½fl oz) white wine
90g (3¼oz) sun-dried tomatoes,
   drained and chopped
15g (½oz) Parmesan or vegetarian
   Italian-style hard cheese,
   grated
70g (2½oz) soft goat's cheese
2 tablespoons finely chopped
   fresh parsley

Place a large pan over a medium heat and add the rapeseed oil. Add the onions and garlic and stir, then cook for 10 minutes, stirring occasionally.

Add the balsamic vinegar and cook for another 20 minutes, stirring occasionally (if the onions are starting to catch, reduce the heat).

Meanwhile, bring a large pan of water to the boil. Add the spaghetti and cook according to the packet instructions, then drain (remembering to reserve a mugful of the water for later).

Add the mixed herbs and wine to the onions and stir, scraping up any bits on the bottom of the pan. Add the sun-dried tomatoes and give another stir.

Add the onion mix to the drained pasta with the Parmesan and toss to combine, adding a splash of pasta water if needed.

Serve the pasta and crumble over the goat's cheese and parsley.

NOTES

Use a mandolin for the sliced onion, but watch your fingers!

Not a fan of goat's cheese? Soft cheese is fine, or you can leave it out completely if you prefer.

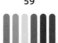

SPINACH & RICOTTA GNUDI

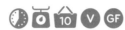

Gnudi, aside from sounding hilarious, are little dumplings in much the same vein as gnocchi (which we will cheerfully eat all day long), but thanks to the ricotta they are that little bit lighter. We have omitted the traditional semolina here, because semolina reminds us of those awful school desserts where you'd be forgiven for wondering if they'd got the canteen and art class supplies mixed up. As a result, the gnudi may not be as firm as you'd like (listen, it happens to us all as we get older) but the end dish is still a treasure.

Go all in on the cherry tomatoes too: mix up the colours and flavours and you'll be rewarded with a treat for the eyes as well as your belly.

SERVES: 4
PREP: 15 minutes
COOK: 40 minutes
CALORIES: 346

500g (1lb 2oz) baby spinach
4 cloves of garlic, crushed
    or grated
300g (10½oz) cherry tomatoes
1 teaspoon sugar
1 teaspoon dried oregano
¼ teaspoon dried chilli flakes
400g (14oz) ricotta
100g (3½oz) soft goat's cheese
65g (2½oz) Parmesan or
    vegetarian Italian-style hard
    cheese, grated
salt and black pepper

Preheat the oven to 180°C fan/400°F/gas mark 6.

Place a large frying pan over a medium heat and spray with a little oil. Add the spinach and half the garlic and cook until wilted.

Spoon the wilted spinach and garlic on to a plate and set aside.

Spray the pan with a little more oil, put back over the heat, and add the rest of the garlic. Cook for 1 minute, then add the cherry tomatoes, sugar, oregano and chilli flakes, and cook for 10 minutes, stirring occasionally.

Roughly chop the cooked spinach and place it in a bowl. Add the ricotta, goat's cheese, two-thirds of the Parmesan and a pinch of salt and pepper, and mix well.

Divide the mixture into 12 equal pieces and roll them into dumpling-shaped balls.

Place the gnudi in a large casserole dish and pour over the cooked tomatoes. Sprinkle with the remaining Parmesan and bake in the oven for 25 minutes.

NOTES

Not a fan of goat's cheese? You can use all ricotta instead if you prefer. We won't judge!

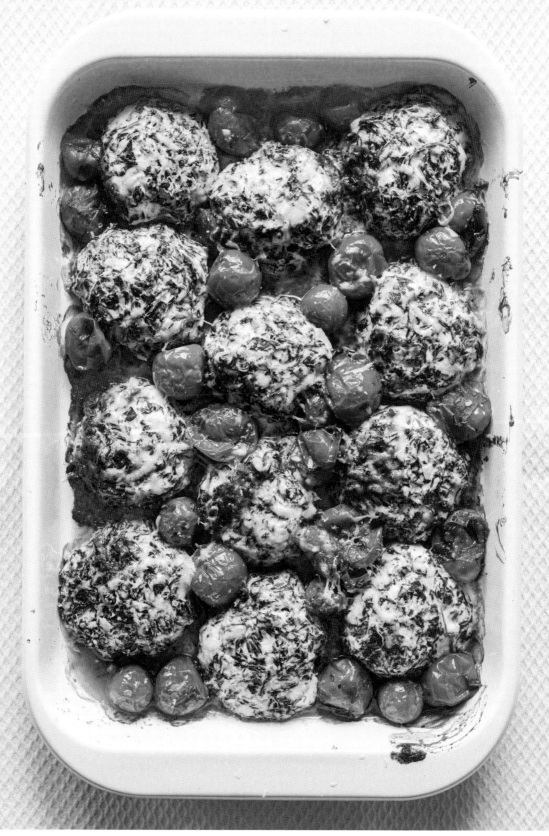

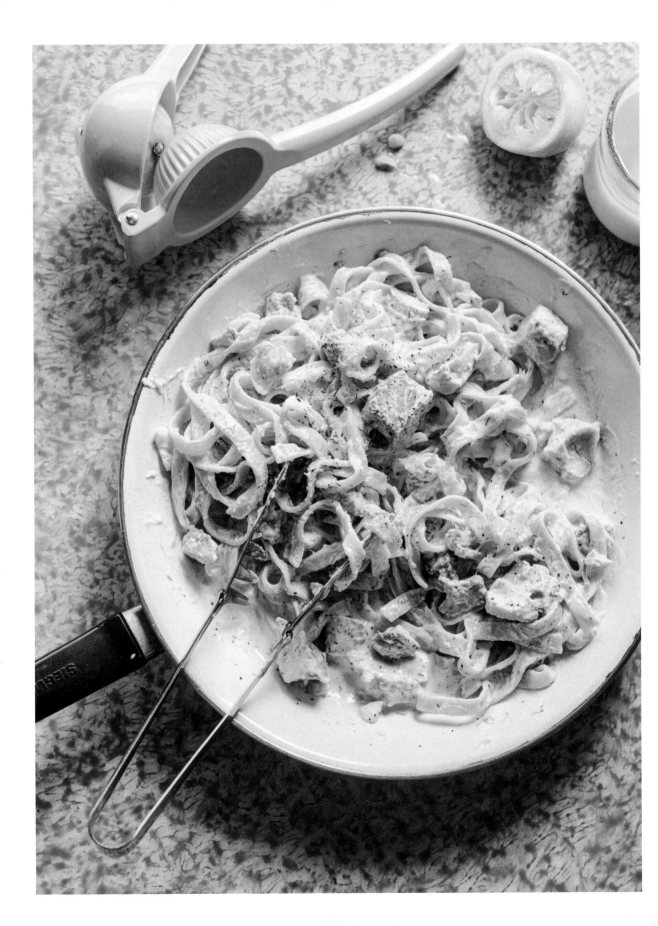

SUPER SPEEDY SALMON TAGLIATELLE

Don't like fish? Hold on a second before flipping the page: nor do we, on the whole, but this recipe somehow transcends our dislike and has become a firm favourite. The key is salmon as fresh as you can get – good fish shouldn't taste fishy, for the most part. That said, if you can't stomach it, swap it out for cooked chicken and no one will ever know.

Paul doesn't suffer the same way I do with fish, though. At distressingly regular points in my childhood my father would bundle us into the car, drive us to some windswept cove in A*se-End, Nowhere and give us an eight-hour lesson in sitting looking listlessly at the sea and smoking. I'm sure there's something therapeutic and wonderful about the practice of fishing, and hey, if it wriggles your line then more power to you, but the only thing we ever caught was pneumonia. You're laughing, but my sister spent four years on an iron lung after my dad was given a new rod for Christmas and took us to Craster after Christmas dinner to try it out. Poor lass, she still whistles like a kettle when she climbs a flight of stairs.

Anyway, the recipe! Do try it. Trust your Cubs.

SERVES: 4
PREP: 5 minutes
COOK: 15 minutes
CALORIES: 499

350g (12oz) tagliatelle
230g (8¼oz) skinless salmon
   fillets, chopped into small
   pieces
3 cloves of garlic, crushed
   or grated
180g (6oz) reduced-fat crème
   fraîche
75g (2½oz) low-fat soft cheese
juice of 1 lemon
15g (½oz) Parmesan cheese,
   grated
¼ teaspoon salt
¼ teaspoon black pepper
1 teaspoon dried dill

Bring a large pan of salted water to the boil. Add the pasta and cook according to the packet instructions, then drain (remembering to reserve half a mugful of the water for later) and put back into the pan, with the lid on.

Spray a large pan with a little oil and place over a medium heat. Add the salmon and garlic and cook for 1 minute.

Add the crème fraîche, soft cheese, lemon juice, Parmesan, salt and pepper, and add a little pasta water, if needed.

Add the drained pasta and stir well to combine for a couple of minutes.

Serve, sprinkled with the dill.

NOTES

As always, any pasta will do!

The sauce will only take a few minutes to make, and will be best as fresh as possible, so only start to cook it once the pasta is ready.

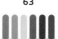

PARMA HAM & LEMON RICOTTA LINGUINI

Ricotta and Parma ham in one delicious, cheesy dish: there's not an awful amount to be said to make this dish seem any more appetising, so instead, I shall confess: I'm only a recent convert to Parma ham. As confessions go that's not exactly up there with an adulterous admission or owning up to the BrinksMat robbery, but hear me out. Those with an active imagination may decide to skip the next paragraph lest the descriptions make you gip.

I'm by no means a fussy eater – you don't get to the state where you need a sit down to catch your breath after brushing your teeth by being picky with calories, after all – but there are certain foods that I struggle to divorce from the mental association in my mind. Parma ham, lying betwixt its greaseproof papers, looks to me like something that might drop off a chemical burn. Roquefort cheese, although utterly heavenly in cooking, makes me think of Paul's feet, both in smell and texture. Cinnamon is another: yes, it can make a dish purr, but it also smells like that overpowering guff that envelops you when you walk into a garden centre at Christmas. And what is a pear if not an apple with the joy removed and bitterness substituted? Never, ever eat pears!

But still we persevere, and so must you, for this is a meal of the ages.

SERVES: 4
PREP: 10 minutes
COOK: 25 minutes
CALORIES: 479

6 slices of Parma ham
250g (9oz) ricotta
2 tablespoons grated Parmesan cheese
zest and juice of 1 lemon
¼ teaspoon black pepper
400g (14oz) linguini
1 handful of rocket

Preheat the oven to 200°C/425°F/gas mark 7.

Line a baking sheet with greaseproof paper (or foil). Roll up the slices of ham and put them on the baking sheet. Cook in the oven for about 10 minutes, then remove and roughly chop.

Meanwhile, mix together the ricotta, Parmesan, lemon zest, 3 tablespoons of lemon juice and the pepper in a bowl.

Bring a large pan of water to the boil and cook the pasta according to the instructions, then drain (reserving half a mugful of the water for later).

Once drained, put the pasta back into the pan. Add the ricotta mixture and toss well to coat – add a little pasta water if needed.

Add the Parma ham and the rocket and give a good stir, then serve.

NOTE

We used linguini for this but really, any pasta is absolutely fine.

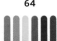

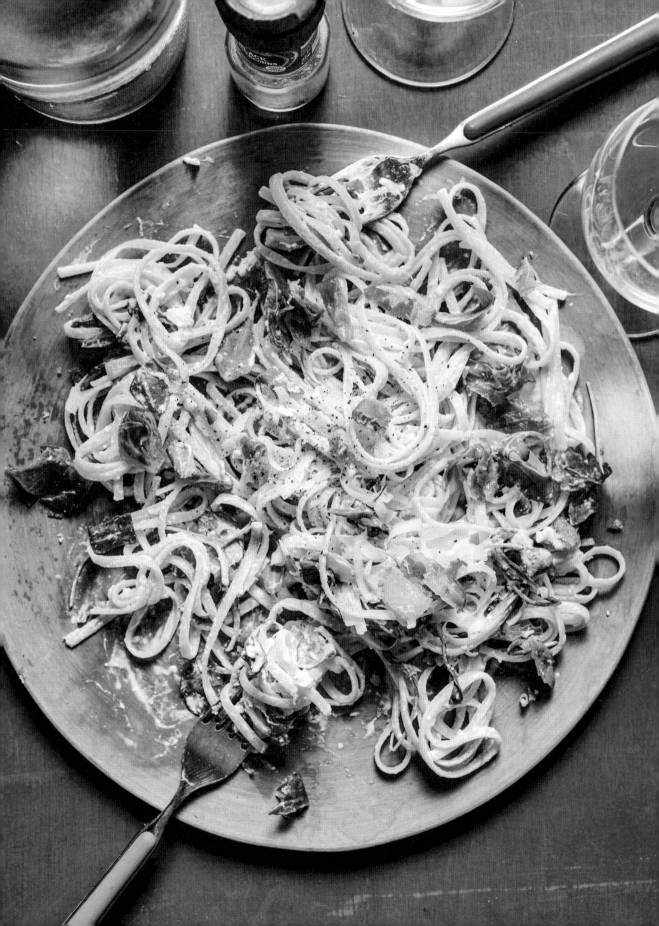

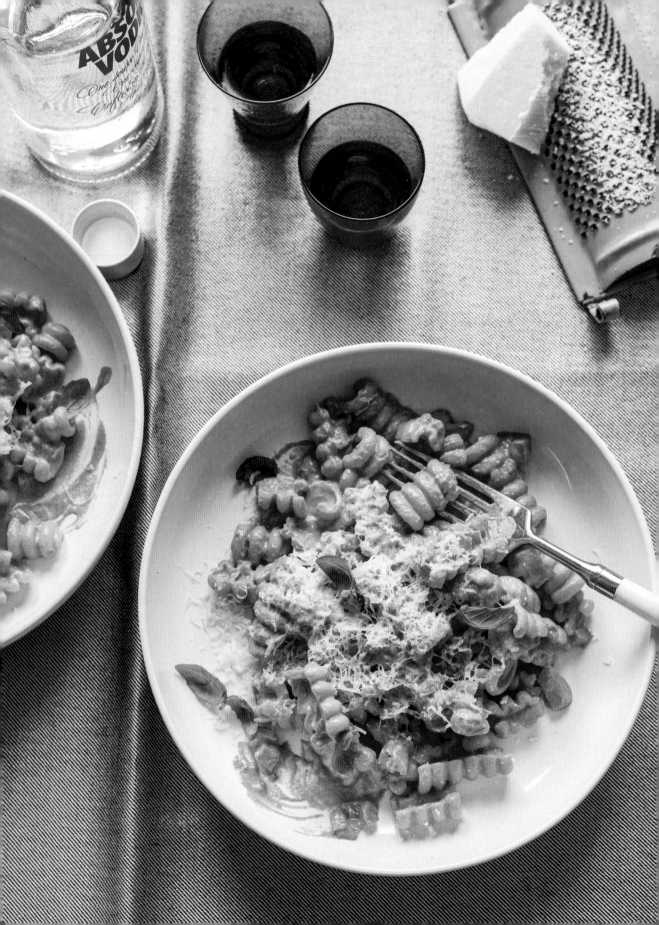

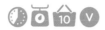

MAMMY'S SPECIAL PASTA

We're calling this pasta 'Mammy's Special Pasta' for the simple reason that it contains hard liquor and so does my mother: it's a tribute to her. Using the same logic, should we ever come up with a recipe that contains 60 car-boot-sale Sterling Superkings, methylated spirits and a lax attitude to the wellbeing of their more successful crotchfruit, we'll name it after Paul's mother.

Of course, you can cheerfully leave the vodka out of this meal and have a thoroughly pleasant time, but you could also leave your socks on during intercourse to keep your feet warm: doesn't mean you should. We are always going to be fans of any dish where we can carouse around the kitchen half-cut while we wait for the pasta to boil. It's either that or make polite conversation, after all, and that's never going to happen at Chubby Towers.

SERVES: 4
PREP: 5 minutes
COOK: 35 minutes
CALORIES: 496

400g (14oz) pasta
1 onion, finely diced
4 cloves of garlic, crushed
    or grated
5 tablespoons tomato purée
½ teaspoon dried chilli flakes
2 shots of vodka
150g (5½oz) low-fat soft cheese
2 tablespoons grated Parmesan
    or vegetarian Italian-style hard
    cheese
5–6 fresh basil leaves, chopped

Bring a large pan of water to the boil and cook the pasta according to the instructions, remembering to reserve a mugful of the water for later, before draining.

Meanwhile, spray a large frying pan with a little oil and place over a medium heat. Add the onion and garlic and cook for about 4 minutes, stirring continuously.

Add the tomato purée, chilli flakes and vodka and cook for another 3–4 minutes, stirring occasionally.

Add about half the mug of pasta water to the pan and stir until smooth.

Bring the sauce to a simmer and stir in the soft cheese, then remove from the heat.

Add the pasta and stir gently until well coated. Add a little more pasta water if needed.

Serve the pasta, sprinkled with the Parmesan and basil.

NOTES

Your kids shouldn't get pissed off with this, but if you really need to, simply leave out the vodka – it's still a very decent pasta dish without it!

Any pasta of your choice will work with this.

SWISS MACARONI & CHEESE

Macaroni cheese, and almost all variants thereof, would absolutely feature on my 'final meal' list. Paul and I were lucky enough to see the always terrific Jay Rayner's tour 'My Last Supper' a couple of years ago, where he discussed, at length and with hilarity, every part of his final meal. You would expect a food writer's last meal to be full of exotic ingredients and frou-frou-ness, but he endeared himself to me immediately by including chips. That's the way to approach it: plenty of stodge, plenty of tasty carbs, plenty of things that would ordinarily make your hips jiggle and your belt groan, but this time it matters not a jot because you'll be dead in a matter of moments.

Now, readers, we ought to make it clear: we aren't pushing you to pop yourselves off after this meal because that simply wouldn't do. But simply, if we are including a dish that we would happily eat before the sweet release (Paul) / terrifying void (James) of death, you know it's good.

Plus, this has apples in it. Apples. In a macaroni cheese. Nope, trust us.

SERVES: 4
PREP: 10 minutes
COOK: 1 hour 15 minutes
CALORIES: 499

4 bacon medallions, finely diced
2 tablespoons butter
2 onions, halved and finely sliced
3 apples, cored and peeled
250g (9oz) potatoes, peeled and cut into 2cm (¾ inch) cubes
225g (8oz) macaroni
120g (4½oz) low-fat soft cheese
50g (1¾oz) Gruyère cheese, grated
¼ teaspoon salt

NOTES

We used Gruyère as it's a traditional Swiss cheese, but Cheddar is absolutely fine too.

Don't be put off by the apple sauce – it's worth it.

We love that this is a Swiss recipe – it's a big plus.

Spray a frying pan with a little oil and place over a high heat. Add the bacon medallions to the pan and cook for 7–8 minutes, until crispy, then set aside.

Spray the frying pan with a bit more oil, place back over a medium-low heat and add the butter. When it's melted, add the onions, sprinkle with a bit of salt and cook for about 30 minutes, stirring occasionally, until golden, then set aside.

Cut the apples into 2cm (¾ inch) cubes. Put them into a saucepan along with 60ml (2fl oz) of water and bring to a simmer over a medium-low heat, stirring occasionally, for about 20 minutes, then mash until smooth and set aside.

Fill a large pan with water and add the potatoes. Bring to the boil over a high heat, add the pasta and cook for about 10 minutes, then drain.

Return the pasta and potatoes to the pan. Add the soft cheese and grated Gruyère, then stir through the caramelised onion and bacon until the cheese has melted.

Serve the pasta on plates and top with the apple sauce.

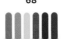

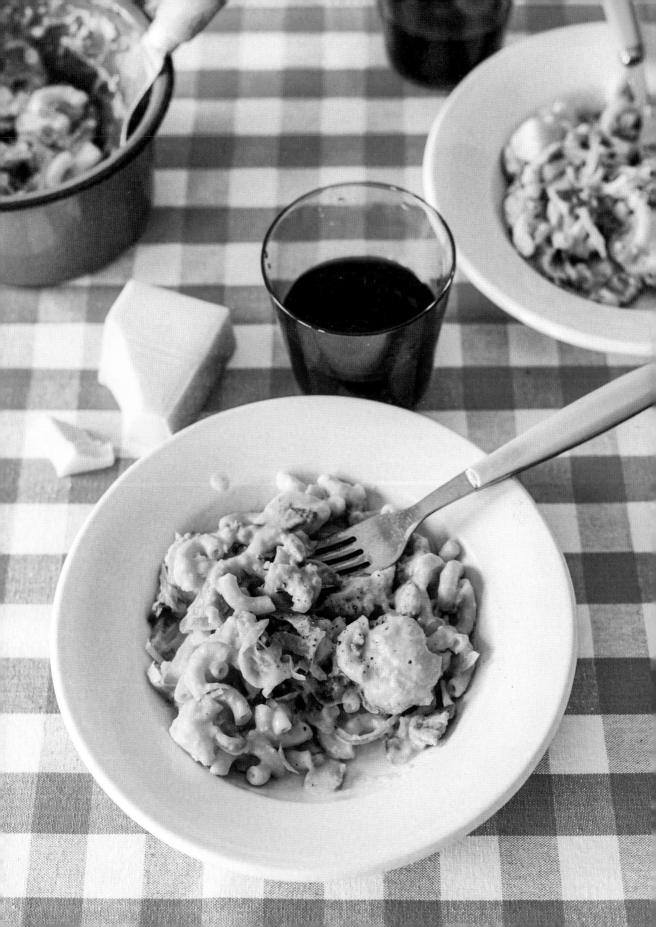

PASTA & SAUCE

Back in the giddy, Quark-scented days when we followed a particular universe of slimming (wink wink) diet plan, one of our favourite meals was one of those packets of 'pasta and sauce' made up with extra cheese added, served atop a steaming pile of chips coated with garlic powder. Looking back, it wasn't the most healthy of choices – we may as well have served it alongside a potato milkshake to complete the carb overload – but it was 'free' and therefore perfectly acceptable.

But we shan't lie: if you're after a carb overload, it's a delicious meal. See the notes if you want to make your own garlic chips, but don't blame us if no one wants to kiss you after. In memory of that dish, we've replicated the best way we can two of the most popular flavours and gussied them up a little. Because it's us, and we're nothing if not fancy terrors. You don't need to serve this with anything other than a smile on your chops. Makes enough for two massive portions and the calorie count is for the base recipe only.

SERVES: 4
PREP: 5 minutes
COOK: 20 minutes
CALORIES: 498

325g (11½oz) conchiglie pasta (any pasta is fine. We use conchiglie because it sounds like a cat sneezing)
1 fat little onion, chopped very finely
350ml (12fl oz) stock, made from a good-quality vegetable stock cube
220ml (7½fl oz) reduced-fat crème fraîche
100g (3½oz) extra strong mature Cheddar cheese, grated

For the cheese and ham
180g (6oz) shredded ham hock (available in most supermarkets, or dice up some ham)
1 teaspoon mustard

For the cheese and broccoli
a few broccoli florets, finely chopped

Cook the pasta in a big pan of salted water, then drain and set aside.

In a frying pan, gently fry the onion until golden. Add the stock and bring to the boil, adding the broccoli here if using.

Lower the heat to medium and stir in the crème fraîche and the cheese, and keep stirring, adding the ham and mustard if using.

When thickened, mix with the pasta and serve.

NOTES

We use an air-fryer for our chips because *of course we do*, but you can also make them on an oven tray – simply cut your potatoes into chips, shake them in a bowl with a good glug of oil and a crumbled beef stock cube, then sprinkle a quarter-tonne (adjust for flavour) of garlic salt over the top of them. Cook them in the oven at 200°C fan/425°F/gas mark 7 for 30 minutes, turning halfway.

We don't normally advocate reduced-fat anything, but you're fine here – the added cheese makes up for it – and if you want to lower the calories still further, use ultra low-fat soft cheese.

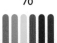

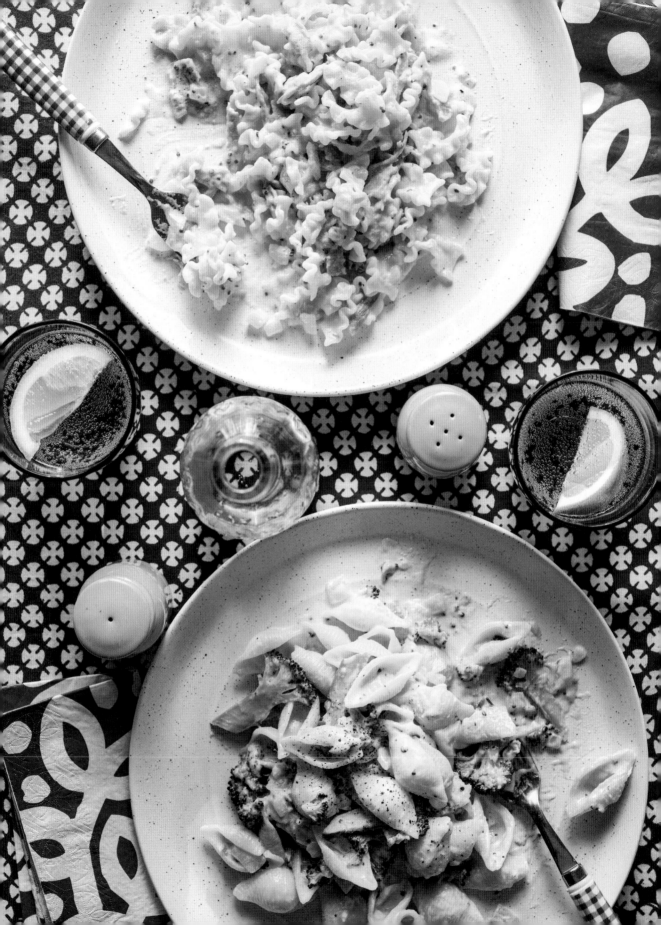

COCONUT LIME CHICKEN PASTA

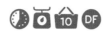

Although this book is us providing you satisfaction in the evenings with our wonderful meals, nearly all of them lend themselves to leftovers being hungrily snaffled the next day for lunch: and none more so than this. It is a very simple recipe indeed that you could absolutely frou-frou up with all sorts of additions, but in all honesty, it doesn't require it.

You must not be tempted to use anything other than coconut milk, though. This is an oft-repeated warning of ours and yet still not a night goes by where I don't stare thin-lipped and utterly furious at our Instagram and spot that someone has skimped and used some awful alternative. You mustn't. We ask so little, and the flavours make it all so worthwhile.

SERVES: 4
PREP: 10 minutes
COOK: 30 minutes
CALORIES: 500

1 × 400ml (14fl oz) tin of light coconut milk
juice of 1 lime
1 chicken stock cube, crumbled
1–2 cloves of garlic, crushed or grated
¼ teaspoon black pepper
2 large skinless, boneless chicken breasts
340g (12oz) spaghetti
2 tablespoons chopped fresh coriander leaves
lime wedges (optional), to serve

In a jug, mix together the coconut milk, lime juice, stock cube, garlic and black pepper and set aside.

Wrap the chicken breasts loosely in cling film and bash with a rolling pin or the bottom of a heavy saucepan until they are an even thickness, about 1½cm.

Bring a large pan of water to the boil. Add the spaghetti and cook according to the packet instructions, then drain and put back into the pan.

Meanwhile, spray a large frying pan with a little oil and place it over a medium-high heat. Add the chicken and cook for 4–5 minutes on each side, then remove to a plate.

Pour the coconut milk mix into the same pan and bring to the boil. Once boiling, reduce the heat to medium-low, put the chicken back into the pan and simmer for 5 minutes.

Remove the chicken from the pan, place on a chopping board and leave to rest. Let the mixture continue to simmer for 5 minutes.

Keep aside 4 tablespoons of the sauce, then pour the rest into the pasta and toss to combine.

Serve the spaghetti on plates, then slice the chicken and place on top. Spoon over the reserved sauce and sprinkle over the coriander. Garnish with lime wedges, if liked.

NOTE

As always with us, any pasta will do!

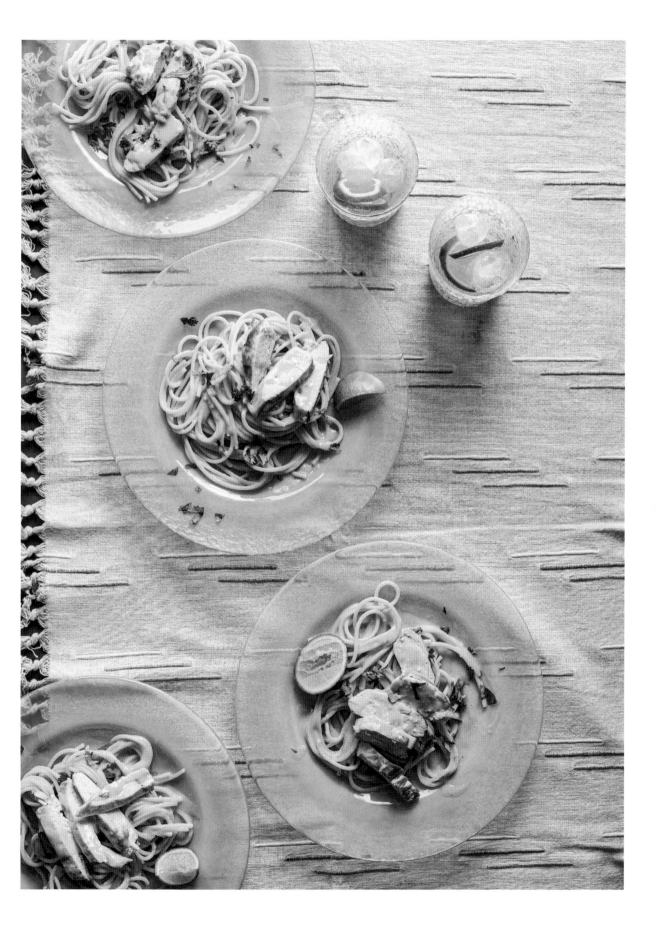

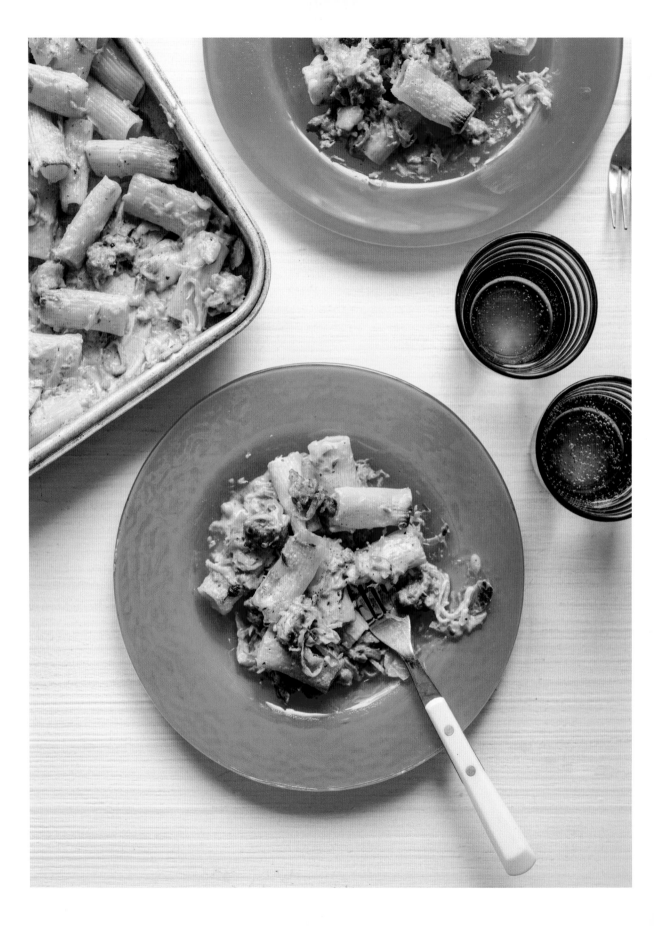

SAUSAGE & SPROUTS

Ah, sprouts. Those who have been with us since the beginning know that this is the next step in our campaign to bring the humble sprout out of the shame cupboard and into the light, so that we can all bask in its tasty, admittedly slightly farty, flavour. We've put them into risotto. We've shredded them into a salad. Now, we're making a pasta dish that you absolutely, utterly must try.

We need you to get behind us on this, and that's not something we usually say. Well no, it is, but it's usually hurriedly barked over our shoulders and certainly not in the context of a sprout recipe. If we can encourage you to put aside your brassicaphobia for an evening and give this a whirl, we believe you will be pleasantly surprised. It's an almost oniony, sausagey delight.

Do it. Come out for the sprout. Of course, if you try it and *don't* like it, you mustn't send us angry letters. We know not what we do.

SERVES: 4
PREP: 10 minutes
COOK: 55 minutes
CALORIES: 500

300g (10½oz) rigatoni
4 pork sausages, skins removed
1 onion, sliced
150g (5½oz) Brussels sprouts, sliced
3 cloves of garlic, crushed or grated
3 teaspoons flour
½ teaspoon fennel seeds
170ml (5¾fl oz) milk
75g (2½oz) low-fat soft cheese
15g (½oz) Parmesan cheese, grated

Bring a large pan of salted water to the boil. Add the pasta and cook according to the packet instructions, then drain, remembering to reserve a mugful of the water for later.

Spray a large frying pan with a little oil and place over a medium-high heat. Add the sausages and onion, stirring frequently to break them up, cook until browned, then add them to the drained pasta.

Add the sprouts and cook for 4–5 minutes, stirring frequently, until starting to brown, then add a splash of the pasta water.

Add the garlic and flour, stir well and cook for 1 minute, then add another splash of pasta water to loosen. Reduce the heat to medium, add the fennel seeds, milk, soft cheese and the rest of the pasta water, and bring to a simmer. Cook for 5 minutes, stirring frequently.

Add the pasta and sausage to the pan and stir well to combine, then top with the Parmesan cheese and place under a hot grill for 5 minutes, until bubbling.

Serve.

NOTES

You know the score now – any pasta will do!

If you fancy an indulgent finish, top with grated Cheddar before placing under the grill.

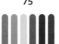

PASTA CASTLE

Forgive my husband this indulgence, please – it's nothing fancy, can be done on the cheap and will make you smile. But enough about Paul. This is a dinner from his childhood, and in a book full of our evening meals, we must allow it. It's also a bloody good pasta dish, and while you don't need to shape it into a castle for the full effect, we are hardly going to caution against it.

Can we take a moment to sing the praises of our wonderful props and food stylist? We throw random nonsense like this at them and they come through every single time. Full thanks are at the back, but this does give me an opportunity to reassure you: if your food doesn't look exactly as photogenic as the photos in our book, just remember we have an amazing, wonderfully skilled team making every dish look just so. Your evening meal is there to nourish you, not to impress your friends and family, after all! So never feel terrible for slopping your portion on a plate and chowing straight down: that's what good food is all about!

That said, if you do make a pasta castle, we absolutely want to see it, so make sure you tag us in on social media!

SERVES: 4
PREP: 15 minutes
COOK: 1 hour 30 minutes
CALORIES: 395

200g (7oz) conchiglie pasta
2 tablespoons butter
2 onions, finely diced
2 cloves of garlic, crushed
300g (10½oz) lean minced beef
100g (3½oz) mushrooms, finely diced
1 × 400g (14oz) tin of chopped tomatoes
400ml (14fl oz) beef stock
500g (1lb 2oz) spinach

Preheat the oven to 180°C fan/400°F/gas mark 6.

Cook the pasta according to the packet instructions, then drain, toss with the butter and mix well. Using a spatula, pack the pasta around the bottom and sides of an ovenproof pudding basin.

Spray a large frying pan with a little oil and place over a medium-high heat. Add the onion and garlic and cook for 2–3 minutes, until softened.

Add the beef mince and mushrooms and cook until browned. Add the tomatoes and beef stock, bring to the boil, then simmer for 30 minutes.

Meanwhile, place a saucepan over a medium heat and add the spinach a handful at a time, stirring gently until wilted.

Pack alternate layers of spinach and mince into the basin and cover with foil. Keep a little of the mince aside for decoration later.

Bake in the oven for 45 minutes. Towards the end of the time, bring the rest of the mince to a simmer.

Gently tip the bowl on to a plate so that it resembles a shit sandcastle, and spoon the reserved mince on top.

NOTE

Yeah, we know, but it's worth it if only for the retro-ness of it.

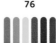

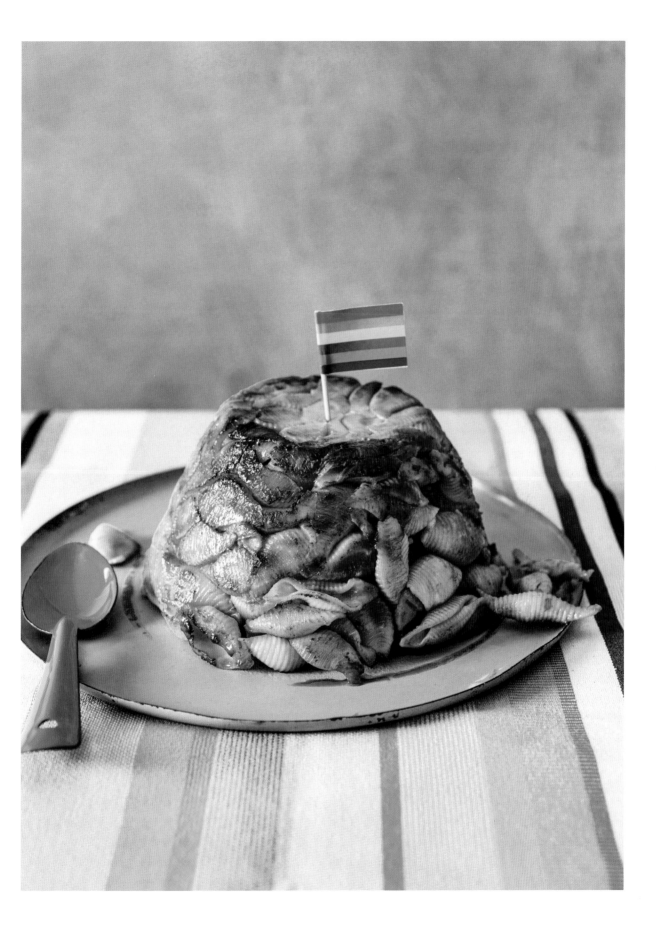

IT'S PUTTANESCA, CHICK xx

I can't say for absolute certain, but I'm sure Paul has called this recipe 'It's Puttanesca, Chick xx' in some weird homage to that Geordie lass who was in *Big Brother 5*, which as references go has to be the most obtuse one yet. I only remember because I was incredibly jealous that she was boffing the one with long hair. He was sharp forgotten about when Anthony turned up in the next series, mind.

Anyhoo. You might look at this puttanesca and dry heave into your elbow at the inclusion of anchovies, and listen, I'm right there with you on this one because goodness, they have no place in a civilised society. But check the notes: we have you covered. That said, Paul had made this a couple of times before I realised anchovies were in it, so please don't fret too much – they don't overpower the dish at all. So, the lesson to be learned here: if your husband is sneaking anchovies into your dinner, that's a ground for divorce recognised by the UK courts.

SERVES: 4
PREP: 5 minutes
COOK: 50 minutes
CALORIES: 469

6 skinless, boneless chicken thighs
6 cloves of garlic, crushed or grated
5 anchovy fillets, finely chopped
¼ teaspoon dried chilli flakes
1 × 400g (14oz) tin of chopped tomatoes
2 tablespoons tomato purée
1 teaspoon dried mixed herbs
90g (3¼oz) pitted mixed olives, chopped
2 tablespoons capers
300g (10½oz) spaghetti
1 tablespoon fresh basil, chopped

Preheat the oven to 200°C fan/425°F/gas mark 7.

Spray a large ovenproof pan with a little oil and place it over a high heat. Add the chicken and cook for about 6–7 minutes, then turn and cook for a further 6–7 minutes. Remove the chicken to a plate.

Reduce the heat to medium, then add the garlic, anchovies and dried chilli flakes and cook for 30 seconds, stirring continuously. Add the chopped tomatoes, tomato purée, mixed herbs, olives and capers, and give it a good stir. Half-fill the empty tomato tin with water, swish about and pour into the pan, then give another stir.

Return the chicken to the pan, then transfer to the oven and cook for 30 minutes.

Meanwhile, bring a large pan of water to the boil. Add the spaghetti and cook according to the packet instructions, then drain, remembering to reserve a mugful of the water for later.

Check the chicken is cooked, and splash in a little of the pasta water if needed.

Serve the chicken with the spaghetti, and sprinkle over the basil.

NOTES

Natch, any pasta will do.

If you don't like anchovies, this is pretty good with diced chorizo instead.

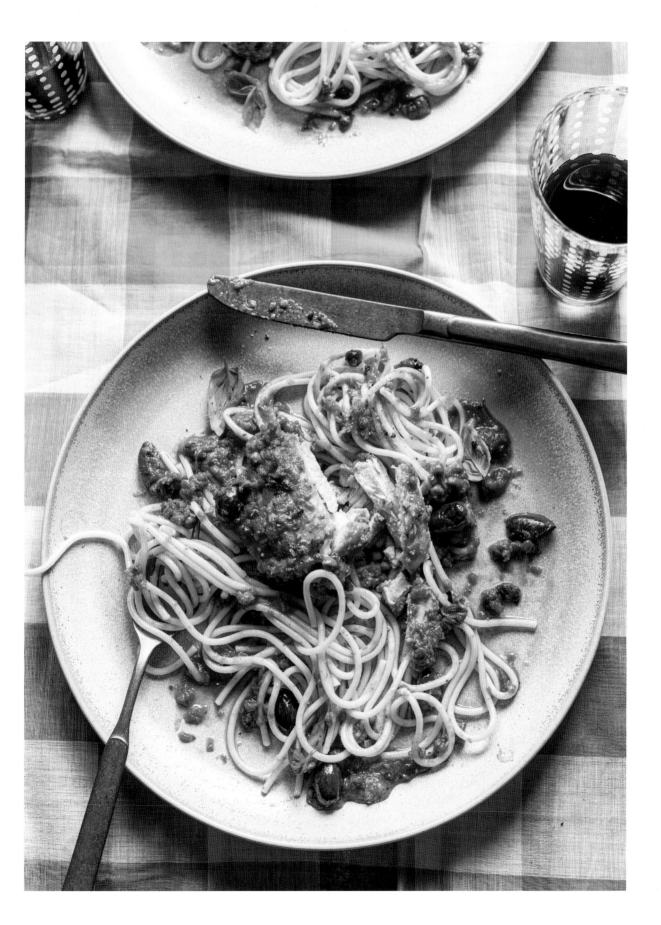

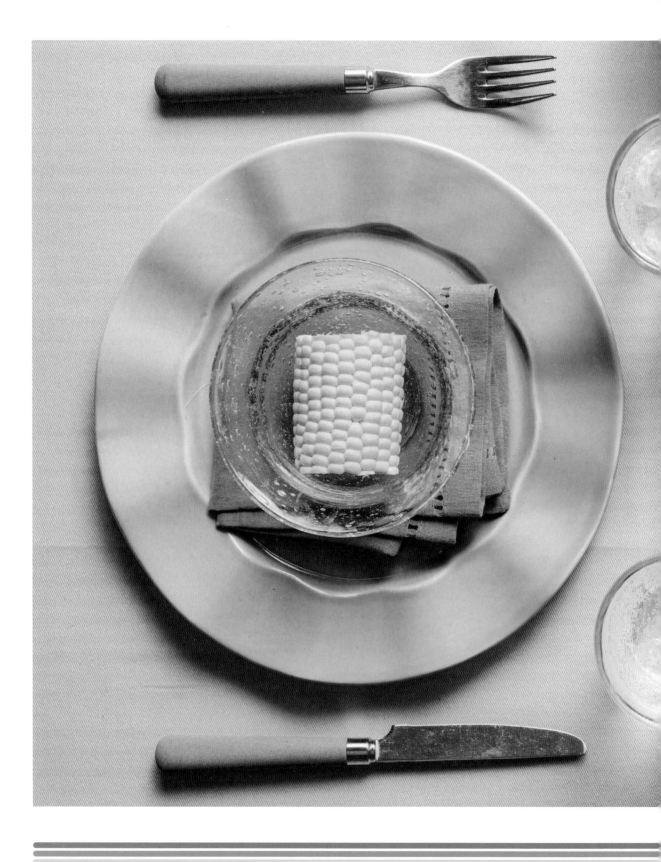

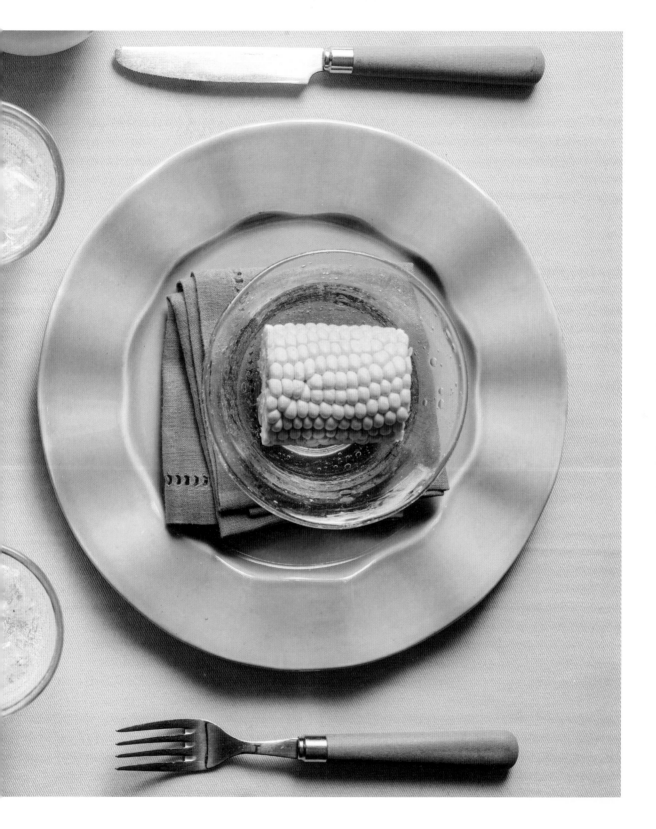

SOUPS, STEWS & CURRIES

SPICY DAHL'S SOUP

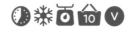

This soup is a homage to a tremendous little lunch I had at the beginning of the year, when I was fortunate enough that Paul allowed me a week away mincing around the North Coast 500, a beautifully scenic road that loops across the top of Scotland. Just me, my car and the overwhelming pressure to be funny on social media. This soup was served up at Ralia Café, just off the A9 on the way to Inverness, and was just the absolute ticket to thaw me from the freezing mountain air. I hope I've done it justice, I do, because the people running the café were unutterably lovely.

That was quite the week, though. I love my husband to bits, I truly do, but there's something about stepping out on your own for a totally unplanned adventure to nourish the soul. It helps, of course, that Scotland is the most magical place, with every turn of that road offering a different, breathtaking vista. I stretched the week out to ten days before I realised I missed Paul's death-rattle snoring and ability to make a room look messy simply by existing and headed home. But I'll say this: a little part of me will always belong to Scotland.

SERVES: 4
PREP: 10 minutes
COOK: 30 minutes
CALORIES: 340

2 onions, peeled and finely diced
2cm (¾ inch) piece of ginger, grated
3 cloves of garlic, crushed or grated
1 tablespoon curry powder
¼ teaspoon smoked paprika
300g (10½oz) red lentils
750ml (28fl oz) vegetable stock
200ml (7fl oz) passata
4 tablespoons fat-free Greek yoghurt
1 red chilli, sliced
handful of coriander leaves

Spray a large pan with a little oil and place over a medium-high heat. Add the onions and cook for 4–5 minutes, stirring occasionally.

Add the ginger and garlic and cook for another minute, then add the curry powder and paprika, and give a good stir.

Add the lentils along with the vegetable stock, and bring to a simmer. Cook for 10 minutes.

Add the passata and simmer for a further 10 minutes.

Serve in bowls, with the Greek yoghurt, sliced chilli and coriander.

NOTE

This is beautiful over some rice!

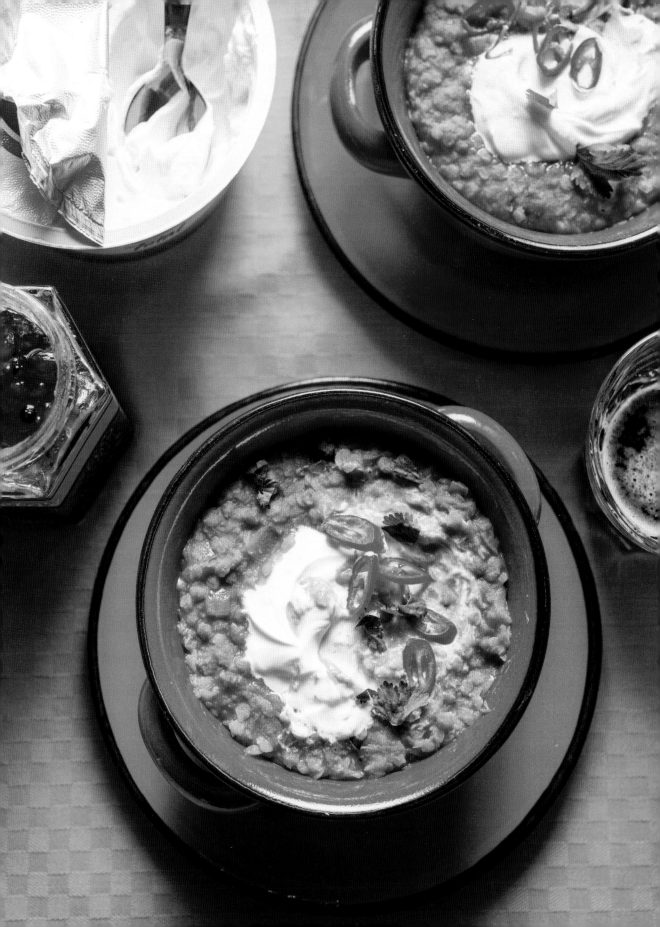

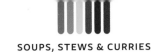
FIVE TASTY SOUPS

There's not room here for a big intro, so we will keep this brief. These soups are terrific, flavourful and bright. Most of them are made with but a few ingredients that you ought to have lolling about in the cupboards and, for an added bonus, they freeze well.

One universal note for all five soups: season as you go. Don't be afraid to add your own touch to the dish – Paul, for example, prefers his food to taste as though someone dredged it from a stormy sea, whereas I'm far more demure. Make these your own!

SPICY RED PEPPER & TOMATO SOUP

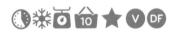

See dish 1, page 86

SERVES: 4
PREP: 10 minutes
COOK: 10 minutes
CALORIES: 63

500g (1lb 2oz) cherry tomatoes, halved
1 jar of roasted red peppers, drained
1 vegetable stock cube
200ml (7fl oz) water
½ teaspoon chilli powder
½ teaspoon paprika
1 teaspoon dried chilli flakes

Blend all the ingredients together.

Pour into a saucepan and warm over a medium-high heat until hot.

SPICY PUMPKIN & BACON SOUP

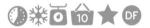

See dish 2, page 86

SERVES: 4
PREP: 10 minutes
COOK: 30 minutes
CALORIES: 109

75g (2½oz) cooked bacon, chopped
500g (1lb 2oz) pumpkin flesh, diced
1 onion, diced
1 teaspoon garlic and ginger paste
500ml (18fl oz) chicken stock
1 teaspoon dried chilli flakes

Set aside a little of the bacon for later, then place all the ingredients in a saucepan and bring to the boil.

Reduce the heat and simmer for 20 minutes, until the pumpkin is soft.

Blend and top with the reserved bacon.

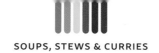
CURRIED CAULIFLOWER SOUP

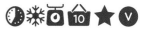

See dish 3, page 86

SERVES: 4
PREP: 10 minutes
COOK: 45 minutes
CALORIES: 97

1 onion, finely diced
1 large cauliflower, cut into florets
3 cloves of garlic, crushed or grated
1 tablespoon hot curry powder

1 litre (1¾ pints) vegetable stock
a splash of Worcestershire sauce
100g (3½oz) fat-free Greek yoghurt

Spray a large pan with oil and place over a medium heat. Add the onion and the cauliflower and cook for 6–7 minutes, until golden.

Add the garlic and curry powder, stir, then cook for 1 minute.

Add the stock and the Worcestershire sauce and bring to the boil, then reduce the heat and simmer for 25 minutes.

Remove from the heat and leave to cool for 5–10 minutes, then stir in the yoghurt and blend.

BORSCHT

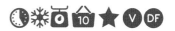

See dish 4, page 87

SERVES: 4
PREP: 10 minutes
COOK: 2 hours 15 minutes
CALORIES: 181

500g (1lb 2oz) beetroot, diced
1 carrot, peeled and diced
1 parsnip, peeled and diced
1 leek, sliced
1 onion, chopped
1.5 litres (2½ pints) vegetable stock
juice of 1 lemon
½ teaspoon grated nutmeg
½ teaspoon ground cinnamon
2 teaspoons dried dill
4 tablespoons crème fraîche

Place all the ingredients, except for the dill and crème fraîche, in a large pan and bring to the boil.

Place a lid on the pan, reduce the heat to low, and simmer for 2 hours.

Remove from the heat and allow to cool for 5–10 minutes, then CAREFULLY blend.

Serve in bowls, with 1 tablespoon of crème fraîche and a sprinkling of dill per bowl.

SUPER SPRING GREENS SOUP

See dish 5, page 87

SERVES: 4
PREP: 10 minutes
COOK: 20 minutes
CALORIES: 67

750ml (1¼ pints) vegetable stock
1 large head of broccoli
200g (7oz) spring greens
100g (3½oz) watercress, or spinach
salt and black pepper

Bring the stock to the boil in a large pan and add the broccoli, spring greens and watercress.

Simmer for 15 minutes, until tender, then add the watercress and use a stick blender to blitz until smooth.

Season with salt and pepper.

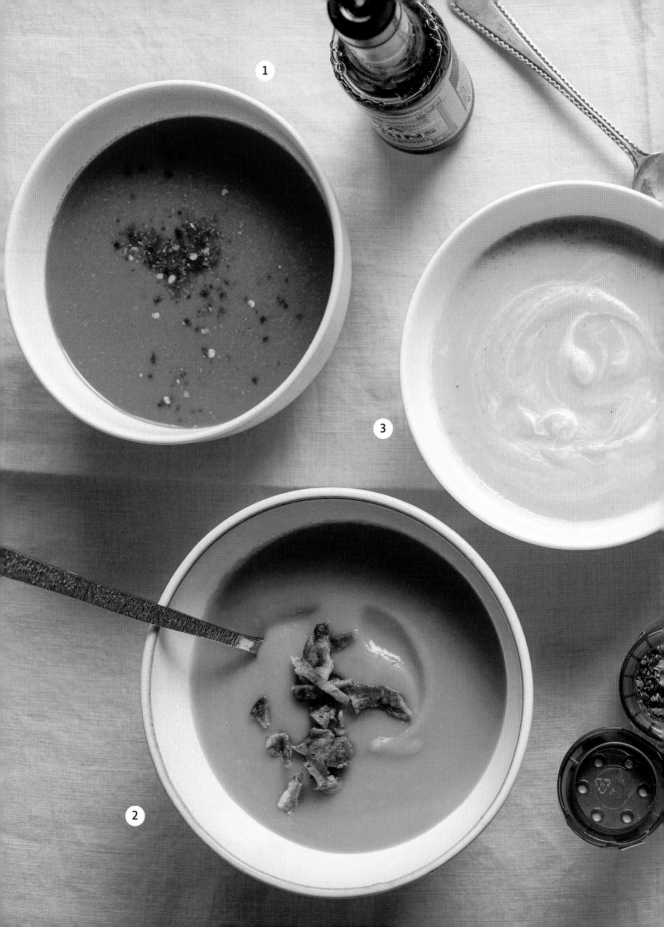

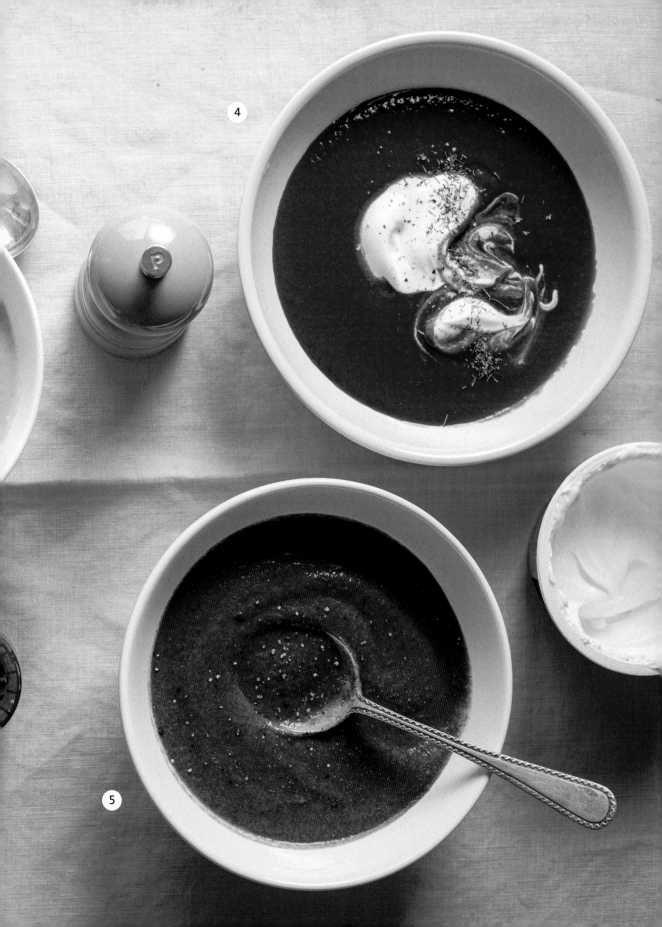

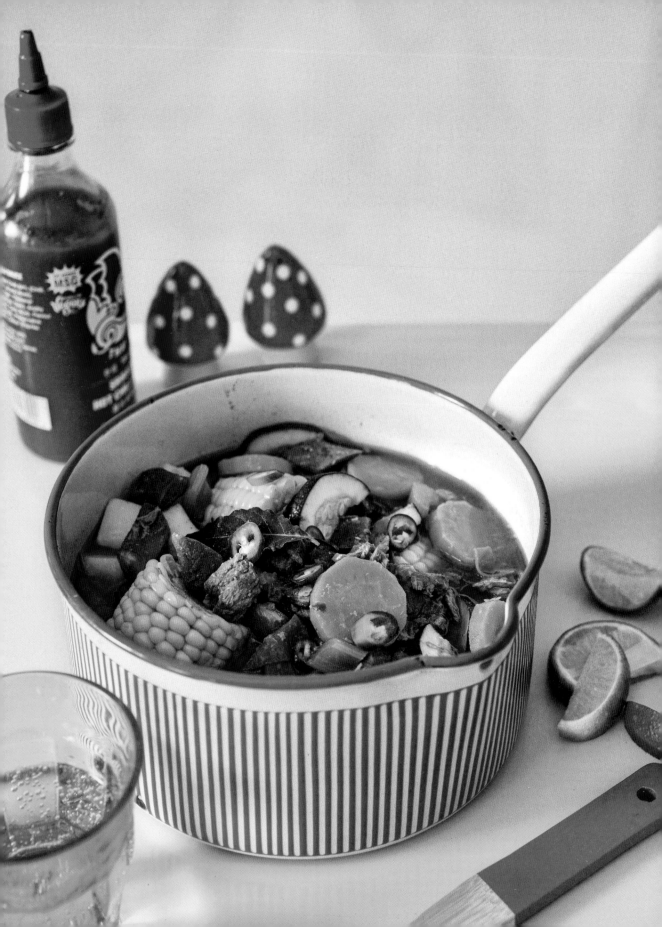

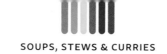
CALDO DE RES

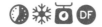

This thick, meaty soup is full of spice and flavour as you would expect from us, with the added benefit of the title looking like an anagram. Perhaps it's my escape-room addled brain, but I look at that, see 'Carlos Edde' and am immediately searching for the next clue.

Have you tried an escape room yet? If not, please make it a thing for the year ahead because they're utterly marvellous. Paul and I have spent over 120 hours being locked in various rooms, solving prison breaks, cowboy mysteries, jewellery heists, Alsatians, the lot. You're not actually locked in and can leave at any time, and they're just so much fun. We've only ever lost one, and in our defence, the instructions were in Icelandic. When the walkie-talkie crackled to life and some guidance was given, it was hard to work out whether the host was steering us to success or choking on a chunk of hangikjöt. We aren't sore at all.

Oh, and unless you're booted through a door by a friend who thinks you're taking too long to climb through, there's no real risk of injury either. Karma caught up with him a few months later when he went clattering over his own legs with an almighty moo, you'll be pleased to know. Anyway, your fabulous soup awaits.

SERVES: 4
PREP: 10 minutes
COOK: 2 hours 25 minutes
CALORIES: 371

500g (1lb 2oz) diced beef
1 onion, chopped
2 large tomatoes, chopped
4 cloves of garlic, crushed
½ teaspoon salt
1 teaspoon cumin
1 teaspoon dried oregano
1 bay leaf
1 beef stock cube, crumbled
½ teaspoon black pepper
2 celery stalks, chopped
2 carrots, sliced
2 potatoes, cut into bite-size
    chunks
2 corn on the cobs, halved
2 courgettes, sliced
200g (7oz) runner beans, trimmed
1 tablespoon sriracha
2 green chillies, sliced
1 lime

Put the beef, onion, tomatoes, garlic, salt, cumin, oregano, bay leaf, beef stock cube and pepper into a large pan and add 1.5 litres (2¾ pints) of water. Bring to the boil, then reduce the heat and simmer for 2 hours.

Add the celery, carrots and potatoes and simmer for another 20 minutes.

Add the corn on the cobs, courgettes and runner beans and cook for another 5 minutes.

Stir in the sriracha, then serve in bowls, topped with the chillies and wedges of lime.

NOTES

This is usually made with oxtail or beef shank, and if you can get your hands on those easily enough, by all means use them instead for a richer flavour. Otherwise, diced beef is fine.

Add more or less sriracha to your liking.

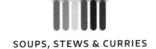
CHICKEN FAJITA SOUP

Before you turn the page with those thin, pursed, disapproving lips at the sight of the long list of ingredients, allow us to throw ourselves at your mercy. Most of the list is spices and herbs that you'll have knocking about, the rest is mainly tins and bits and pieces you'll have in the cupboard. If you trust us enough to take a gamble, you'll be rewarded with a thick, wholesome and tasty soup that'll see you through any evening.

SERVES: 4
PREP: 15 minutes
COOK: 40 minutes
CALORIES: 537

1 onion, finely diced
4 cloves of garlic, crushed
1 red pepper, finely diced
2 teaspoons chilli powder
2 teaspoons smoked paprika
1 teaspoon onion granules
1 teaspoon garlic granules
1 teaspoon ground cumin
1 teaspoon dried oregano
1 litre (1¾ pints) chicken stock
2 × 400g (14oz) tins of chopped
    tomatoes
2 skinless, boneless chicken
    breasts
200g (7oz) low-fat soft cheese
300g (10½oz) tinned sweetcorn,
    drained
1 × 400g (14oz) tin of black beans,
    drained
1 avocado
50g (1¾oz) Cheddar cheese,
    grated
a handful of tortilla chips,
    crushed
a handful of fresh coriander,
    roughly chopped
1 lime, quartered

Spray a large pan with a little oil and place over a medium-high heat. Add the onion, garlic and red pepper and cook for 5 minutes, stirring occasionally.

Add the chilli powder, paprika, onion and garlic granules, cumin and oregano and stir. Add the stock and the chopped tomatoes and stir well.

Add the chicken and bring to the boil, then reduce to a simmer, cover with a lid, and cook for 20 minutes.

Use a slotted spoon to remove the chicken from the pan. Shred with two forks, then return to the pan. Add the soft cheese and stir gently until well combined. Add the sweetcorn and black beans and cook for 3–4 minutes.

Meanwhile, halve the avocado and remove the stone. Scoop out the flesh and dice.

Serve the soup in bowls, topped with the diced avocado, grated cheese, tortilla chips and coriander, with lime quarters on the side for squeezing over.

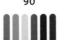

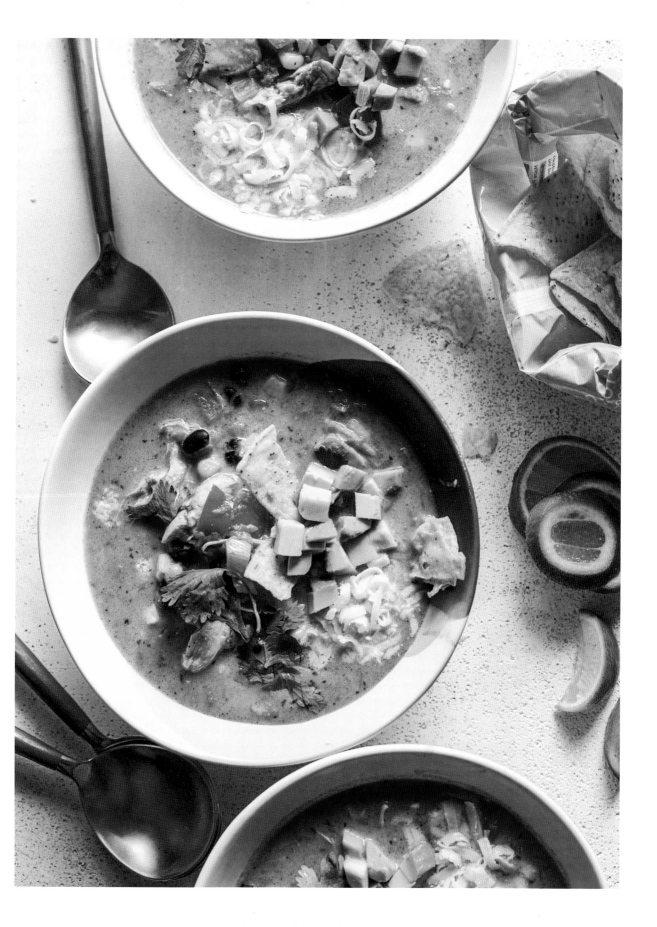

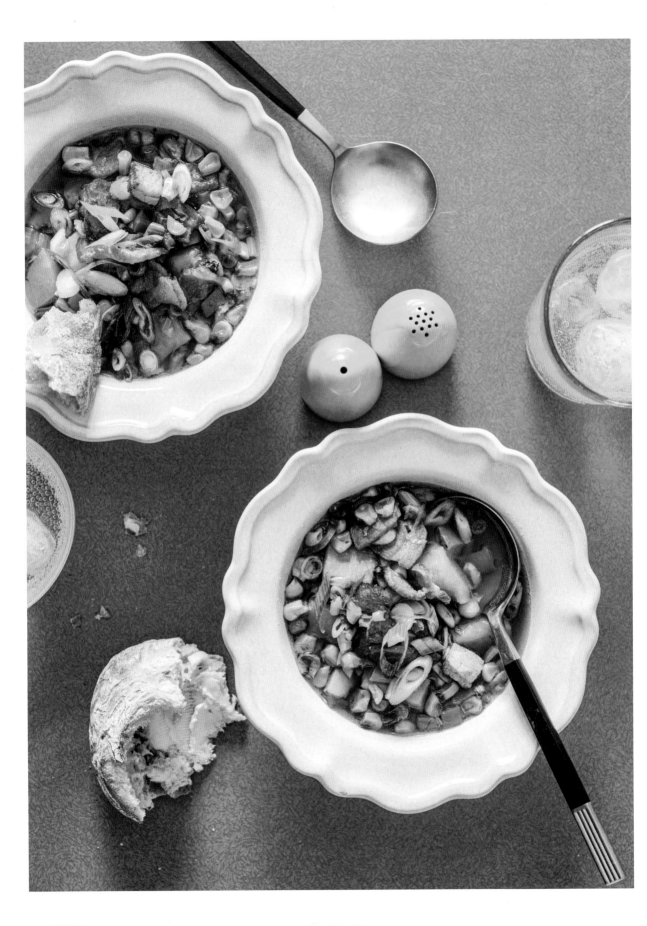

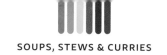
CORN CHOW-DAH!
SAY IT! SAY CHOW-DAH!

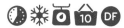

Nothing on this Earth can convince me that we should be eating sweetcorn: it clearly doesn't want to be digested, no matter how hard you try. For years I stuck to this motto and avoided it as best I could, forever scared by the anaemic sweetcorn that you used to get in those awful bags of 'mixed veg'. It tasted of bugger all.

However, like Newton with his apple, I had an epiphany of my very own in a branch of My Thai in Leeds. I was enduring dinner with a friend who, in between spilling *his* dinner all down *my* shirt and spitting while he talked, recommended I tried the corncakes. Well, a bit of his corncakes. Well, no, a tiny bit of the corncakes I'd bought for the table. They were incredible. And so, from that moment on, I vowed to try corn anew.

Paul, inspired by my constant need for attention/new dishes, set about trying to bastardise the smoked fish chowder we'd had previously and pulled together this snappy little number. I love it, and I hope you love it too.

SERVES: 4
PREP: 10 minutes
COOK: 40 minutes
CALORIES: 404

4 corn on the cobs
4 bacon medallions, chopped
2 cloves of garlic, crushed or grated
1 onion, finely diced
1 red pepper, deseeded and finely diced
2 tablespoons flour
1.5 litres (2½ pints) chicken stock
3 potatoes, peeled and diced into 2cm (¾ inch) cubes
1 teaspoon dried thyme
1 teaspoon salt
1 teaspoon black pepper
2 spring onions, finely sliced

Preheat the grill to medium-high. Spray the corn with a little oil, then cook under the grill for about 10 minutes, turning every 2 minutes.

Meanwhile, spray a large saucepan with a little oil and place over a medium-high heat. Add the bacon and cook for 8–10 minutes, until crispy, then remove from the pan and set aside.

Reduce the heat to medium and add the garlic, onion and red pepper. Cook for 3–4 minutes, until the onion has softened and turned translucent.

Sprinkle the flour over the vegetables, stir well and cook for 1 minute. Add the stock and potatoes and stir well.

Meanwhile, slice the corn kernels from the cobs. Set the kernels aside and add the cobs to the pan. Simmer for 10 minutes, then remove the cobs.

Add the corn kernels to the pan, along with the thyme, salt and pepper, and stir well.

Serve the chowder in bowls, topped with the bacon and spring onions.

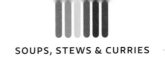
SAUSAGE & KALE SOUP

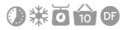

Sausages: we love them, you love them, our dog loves them – but in the interests of doing something different with a sausage (that won't get us done for indecency) we've whacked them into this wonderfully restorative soup.

Yes, our dog. Those poor souls who have been with us since the first book may recall me rather rashly promising Paul that if the book did well and I could work from home, we would get a dog. Naturally I had no intention of following through on this promise, but, with all the devil-may-care attitude of a *Sunday Times* Best-Selling Author (and under the pressure of seeing some cute puppies), I folded like a busker's accordion. As a result, Chubby Towers now has the most ineffectual guard dog you've ever seen in the form of our springer spaniel, Goomba.

He is glorious, because of course he is: we never knew our life was missing something that would become so excited when we return from the bathroom that he pees all over the floor. Every square foot of our carpet is littered with toys, every item of clothing casually covered in white dog hair. For all that I like to pretend that I'm indifferent, I utterly adore him – though I'm never using printed media to make promises ever again.

Well, one more: I promise you'll bloody love this soup. What a segue!

SERVES: 4
PREP: 10 minutes
COOK: 25 minutes
CALORIES: 389

8 thick pork sausages
½ teaspoon fennel seeds
1 onion, diced
3 cloves of garlic, crushed
    or grated
2 potatoes, peeled and diced
½ teaspoon dried mixed herbs
¼ teaspoon dried chilli flakes
1.25 litres (2 pints) chicken stock
140g (5oz) chopped kale

Spray a large saucepan with a little oil and place over a medium-high heat. Add the sausages and cook for 5 minutes, until browned (they don't need to be fully cooked), then remove them to a plate and slice.

Add the fennel seeds to the pan and stir around for a minute or two. Add the onion, garlic, potatoes, mixed herbs and chilli flakes and cook for 5 minutes, stirring occasionally.

Add the stock to the pan along with the sausages and bring to the boil, then reduce to a simmer and cook for another 8 minutes.

Add the kale to the pan and cook for 3–4 minutes until wilted, then serve.

NOTE

Not a fan of kale? Chard, Savoy cabbage and cavolo nero work just as well.

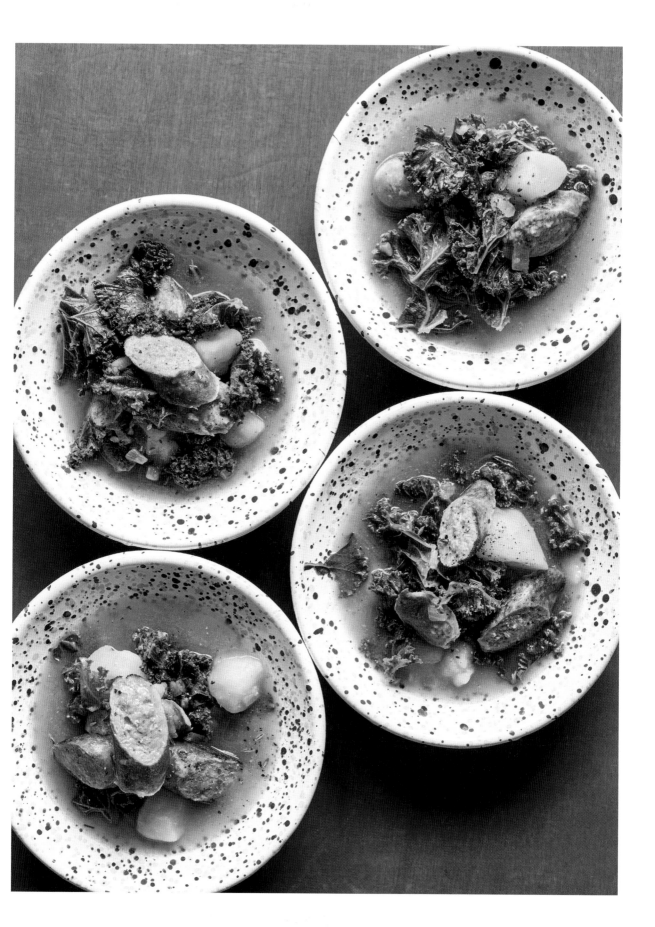

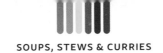

MOREISH CHICKEN

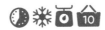

We wanted to rhyme moreish with something else, but our publishers wouldn't let us. Anyway, my mum would have had something to say: she can be quite fussy when it comes to the use of language. She does like to act as an auditor for a lot of my writing, and the number of times I'll wake up to a terse message saying I 'can't use words like that on the Internet' is truly baffling.

While we're on the topic of my mother, I am going to use this space to put something right. Over the course of the last two books I have portrayed my mother as Vera from ITV, a Catherine Cookson tragi-heroine, a filthy lush, all sorts. And yet I've never mentioned in print how much she used to look like Irene from *Home and Away*. You'll see a touch more of this sass in the recipe for Mammy's Special Pasta (page 67).

But no, I'll say this now: I could not hope for better. For all that I do love to take the mick, she (and my dad!) are always there for the both of us and never let us down.

Enough sentimentality, though: this chicken dish deserves your attention. Paul made a note to 'serve with pasta' but the man is a fool – clearly this is made to be sloshed all over spaghetti. And yes, I know that's a pasta, but don't make me send my mother round.

SERVES: 4
PREP: 5 minutes
COOK: 45 minutes
CALORIES: 409

600ml (20fl oz) chicken stock
½ teaspoon mustard powder
½ teaspoon dried thyme
1 teaspoon onion granules
75g (2¾oz) low-fat soft cheese
6 bacon medallions, diced
6 skinless, boneless chicken thighs
2 teaspoons mixed herbs
4 cloves of garlic, crushed or grated
3 tablespoons flour
45g (1½oz) Cheddar cheese, grated
1 bunch of fresh parsley, chopped

In a bowl, whisk together the stock, mustard powder, thyme, onion granules and soft cheese and set aside.

Spray a large saucepan with a little oil and place over a medium-high heat. Add the bacon and cook until crispy, then remove to a plate and set aside.

Open out the chicken thighs, add them to the pan and sprinkle over the mixed herbs. Cook for 5 minutes, then turn and cook for another 5 minutes. Remove the chicken to a plate.

Add the garlic to the pan and stir in the flour, stirring continuously for 1 minute. Add a ladleful of the stock mixture and stir continuously, repeating until all the stock has been added and the sauce is smooth. Bring to the boil, then reduce to a simmer until thickened. Reduce the heat to low and stir in the Cheddar.

Add the chicken and bacon and gently stir until coated, then cover with a lid and simmer for 5 minutes.

Serve with the parsley sprinkled on top.

NOTES

This is lovely with some pasta, or a potato gratin.

If freezing, add the Cheddar when reheating.

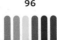

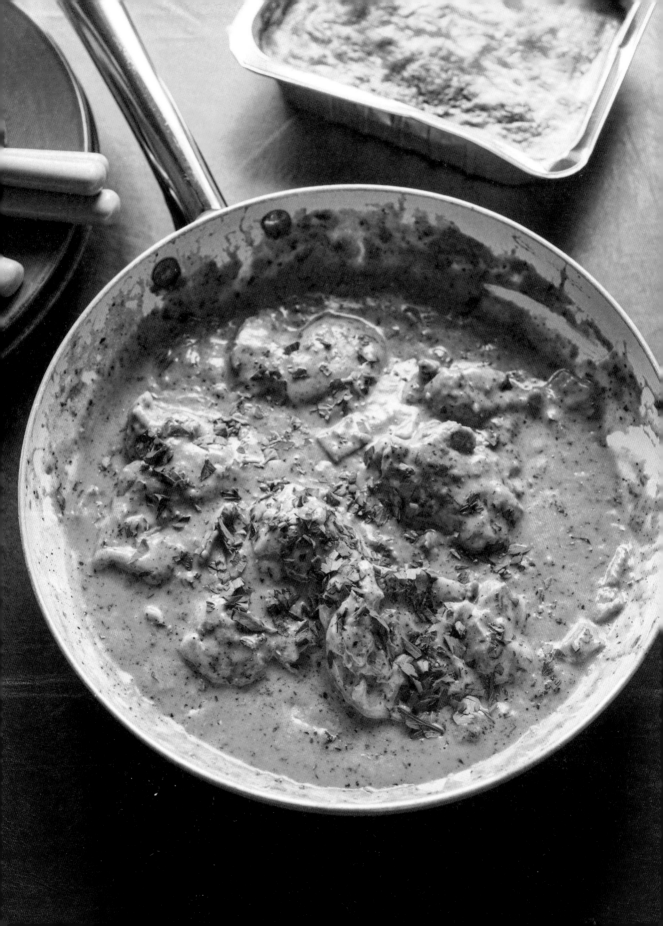

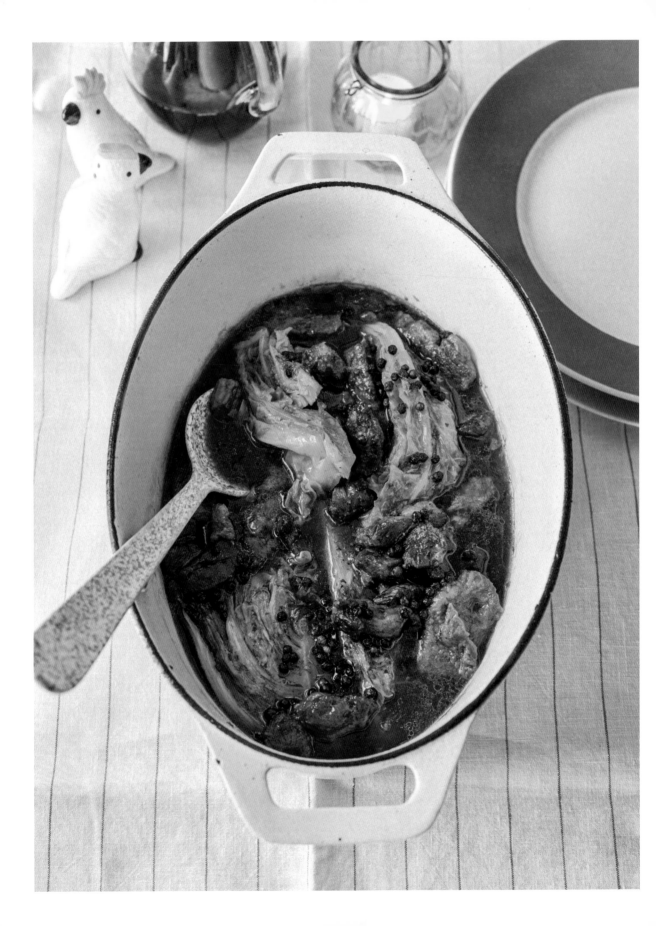

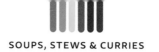
YOU FINK FRANK WANTS STEW?
(MUTTON DRESSED AS LAMB?)

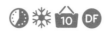

We beg of you: forgive us the *Eastenders* reference. This is a simple lamb stew we tried on our travels, but when we saw that the Norwegians tend to use mutton whereas we have used lamb, all the bits fell into place for the best title yet. For most, the title will mean absolutely nothing and you'll probably assume we've been huffing something we shouldn't (for the most part, that's a safe guess), but for those that know, you'll agree it is glorious.

We begged the publishers to dress us as Pat and Peggy from *Eastenders* and let us replicate their famous scrap for our author photos, but they played a harder game than one might expect given we keep their office Christmas party in name-brand crisps. Nevertheless, it works so well: I would be Pat, the easy-going tart with a propensity towards garish jewellery and bad-choice men. Paul, of course, would be Peggy, simply because he's 4ft 11 in heels. We would throw over our dining table, I'd chuck a glass off the wall and Paul would yell 'NO WONDER WOY CAN'T DO IT' and it would just be *sublime*.

Please, you mustn't be tempted to embellish this recipe. It may look like it won't amount to much, but you need to trust us that the simplicity of the dish is what makes it sing. Oh, and of course, if you can get mutton, do!

SERVES: 4
PREP: 10 minutes
COOK: 3 hours
CALORIES: 463

750g (1lb 10oz) lamb shoulder,
   diced into 2cm (¾ inch) chunks
2 tablespoons flour
3 teaspoons salt
1 sweetheart cabbage
5 tablespoons whole peppercorns
750ml (1¼ pints) vegetable stock

Toss the diced lamb with the flour and salt until well coated.

Slice the cabbage in half lengthways, then widthways into wedges.

Stuff the cabbage into a large pan, and place the lamb and peppercorns on top.

Pour over the vegetable stock and bring to a simmer, then reduce to low and cover with a lid.

Cook for 2–3 hours.

NOTES

Mutton is traditionally used in Fårikål but we've used lamb, as it's easier to find. If you can get mutton, though, give it a go! It's just as tasty!

The beauty of this lies in its simplicity. You might be tempted to throw in extra stuff, but we really recommend trying it as it is first. It's totally worth it.

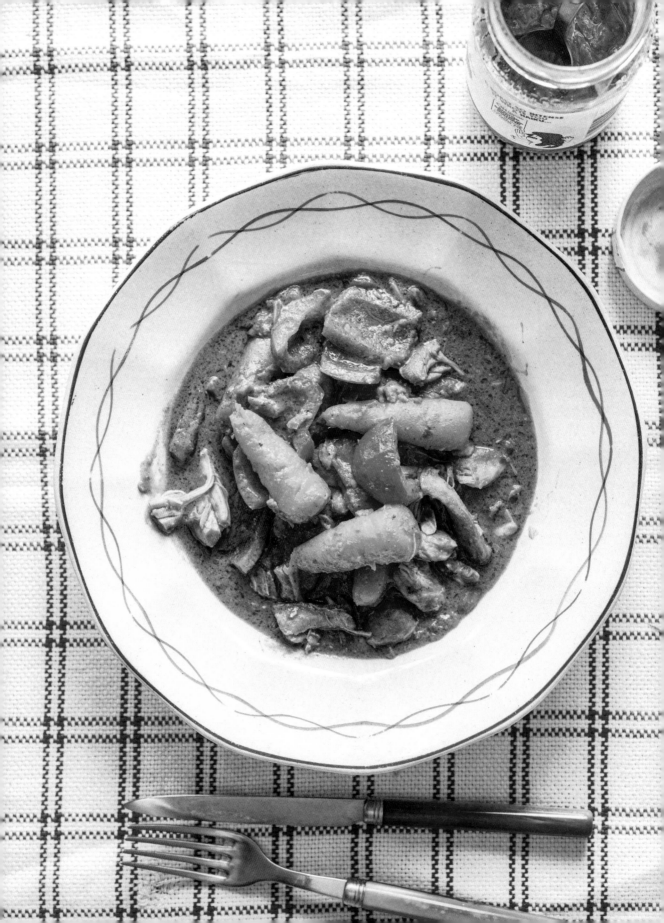

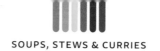
CHICKEN & PEANUT STEW

If you pinned us down (and good luck with that, unless you're planning on hiring a JCB) and demanded we picked one more unusual recipe for you to try, we'd tell you to give this a go.

Slow cooking is terrific if you have the time to let something sit and bubble away for half a day, but it does tend to take away any bite to the food. So, readers, you could absolutely bubble it away on a low simmer for a couple of hours instead if you must.

SERVES: 4
PREP: 10 minutes
COOK: 8 hours
CALORIES: 492

For the marinade
2 cloves of garlic, crushed
1 teaspoon grated root ginger
½ teaspoon fenugreek
½ teaspoon paprika
½ teaspoon salt
½ teaspoon black pepper

For the stew
600g (1lb 5oz) skinless, boneless
    chicken thighs
1 tablespoon grated root ginger
1 green chilli, finely chopped
1 large onion, finely sliced
2 cloves of garlic, crushed
    or grated
10 Chantenay carrots (or any
    baby carrot)
3 tablespoons tomato purée
1 teaspoon paprika
2 teaspoons dried chilli flakes
250ml (9fl oz) passata
600ml (20fl oz) chicken stock
115g (4oz) reduced-fat peanut
    butter
pinch of salt
1 red pepper, deseeded and
    cut into chunks
1 green pepper, deseeded and
    cut into chunks

Put the chicken into a bag and add all the marinade ingredients along with half the ginger and green chilli used for the stew. Shake well to coat, then leave to marinate for 30 minutes.

Spray a large frying pan with a little oil and place over a medium-high heat. Add the chicken and cook for 4–5 minutes each side, then remove to a chopping board and dice into chunks.

Add the onion and garlic to the same pan with the remaining ginger and green chilli and cook for a few minutes, until the onion has started to brown.

Put the chicken into a slow cooker with the onion and add the carrots, tomato purée, paprika, chilli flakes, passata, chicken stock, peanut butter and a pinch of salt. Stir gently to mix everything well.

Cover the pan and cook for 6 hours.

Add the red and green peppers to the pan and cook for another hour, then serve.

NOTES

If your slow cooker has a 'high' setting, you can reduce this down to 4 hours (and add the peppers for the last half an hour).

Chicken breast will work, but as usual, the thighs are always better!

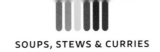
NEAPOLITAN BEEF STEW

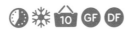

You can't beat a good stew when the nights are closing in (nor can you beat a good Stu when the nights are long), and this is one of those suppers which, once you've done the absolute bare minimum of preparation, you can leave to hubble-bubble on the hob until it's time to serve.

Now, come with me a moment and take a look at the notes below the recipe. Paul has put 'serve with rustic bread'. I have racked my brains (at least, what is left of them after an entire decade eating those Netto bacon grill tins back in the 1990s) and I can't think what he means. Rustic is one of those frightful adjectives that gets used to charmingly elevate a shit-hole barn on Airbnb to something you can justify paying £200 a night for while the rats chew your toenails off.

I'm terribly aware that me taking any sort of stance on frou-frou language is hypocrisy personified, given I write like a 1920s dandy at any given point, but I care not a jot: 'rustic' can get in the bin. Let's speak as we find: gan get yersel' a stottie, pet.

SERVES: 4
PREP: 15 minutes
COOK: 3 hours 20 minutes
CALORIES: 438

1 carrot, peeled and finely diced
1 celery stalk, finely diced
900g (2lb) diced stewing beef
20g (¾oz) fresh parsley, finely
   chopped
2 bay leaves
1kg (2lb 4oz) onions, peeled
   and sliced
175ml (6fl oz) white wine
½ teaspoon dried oregano
½ teaspoon salt
½ teaspoon pepper

Spray a large saucepan with a little oil and place over a medium-high heat. Add the carrot and celery and cook for 3–4 minutes, until softened.

Add the beef and parsley and cook for 5–10 minutes, until the beef is browned.

Add the bay leaves and onions and stir well (don't worry if the pan looks full – it'll reduce down!). Add the wine, oregano, salt and pepper, cover with a lid, and simmer over a low heat for 3 hours, stirring occasionally.

Remove the bay leaves and serve.

NOTES

Don't fret that this looks like it is too dry – that's how it's supposed to be!

This is lovely served with some rustic bread.

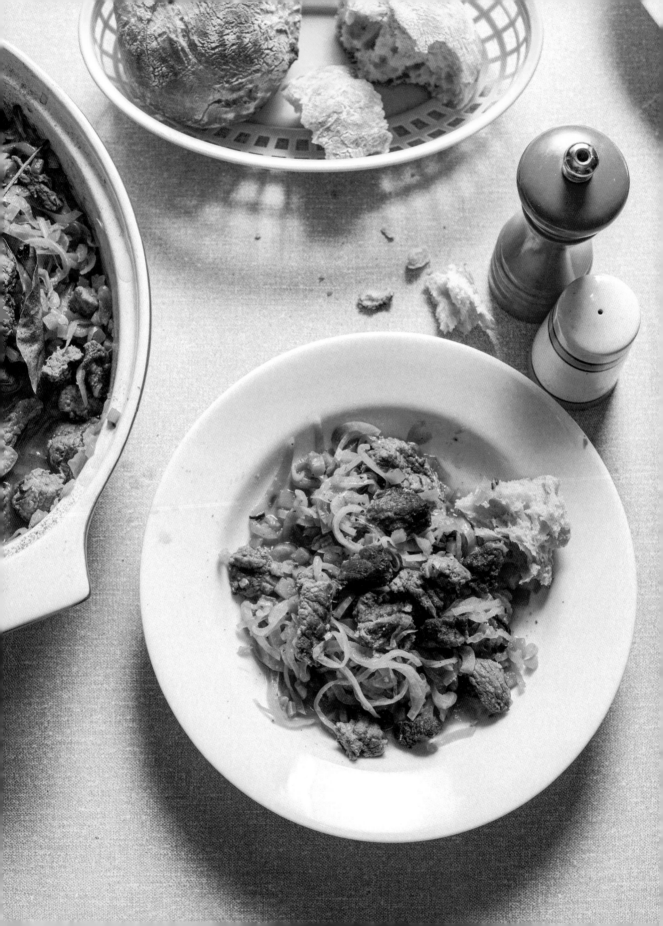

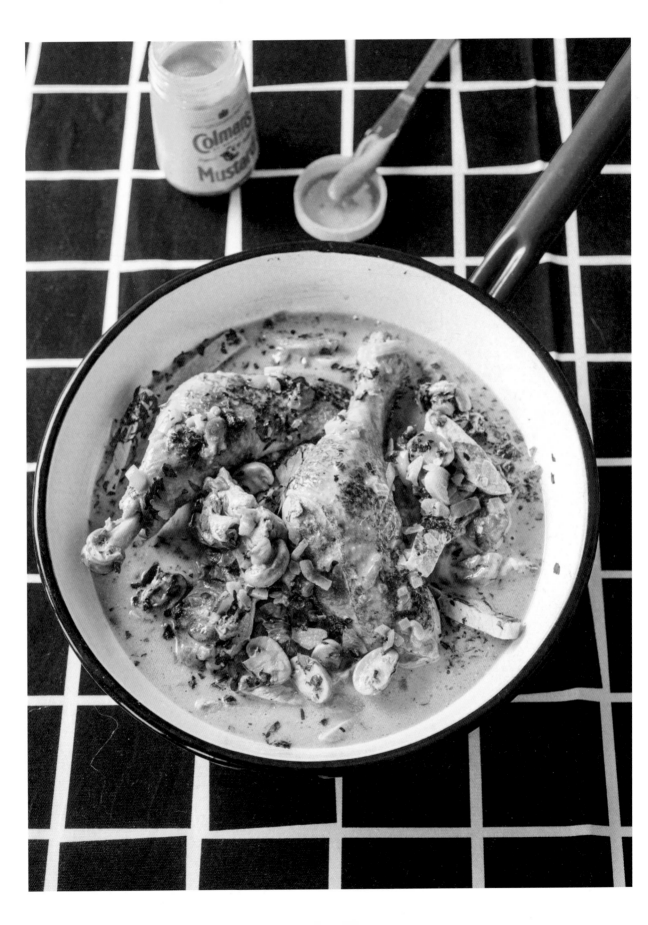

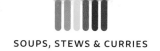
COQ AU VIN BLANC

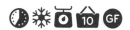

It amazed us that, in the nine years we have been stumbling our way through twochubby-cubs, we have never tried to do a coq au vin recipe. We can shoehorn all manner of innuendo into the most innocent of dishes, but we've never attempted the one meal that sounds like something James would order in a layby. It's beyond us.

Perhaps the reason is we aren't fans of red wine, which is the usual vehicle for this dish. We have tried, we promise, but we can't get away with drinking something that tastes like perfume mixed with diesel. All manner of friends have taken us by the elbow and reassured us that 'we will love it if we just try it', but honestly, no. I can think of only one occasion where I have enjoyed a glass of red wine and I was merrily, merrily intoxicated on all manner of other things at the time: for all I know, it was probably Ribena with some Night Nurse poured in.

So imagine the delight when we realised you don't need red wine at all and it is positively encouraged that you swap it out for white in some places. Some tinkering, some swearing at each other, more trips to buy wine from Londis than can ever be considered decent in one weekend, and we think we nailed it. Purists may disagree, but they can kiss our cheeks.

SERVES: 4
PREP: 10 minutes
COOK: 1 hour 20 minutes
CALORIES: 499

4 bacon medallions
8 chicken pieces (thighs, drumsticks or breasts)
1 onion, finely diced
4 cloves of garlic, thinly sliced
225g (8oz) button mushrooms, halved
500ml (18fl oz) dry white wine
190g (6¾oz) half fat crème fraîche
a bunch of fresh parsley, chopped
salt and black pepper

Spray a large pan with a little oil over a high heat and add the bacon. Cook until crispy, then remove to a plate and roughly chop.

Put the chicken into the pan, sprinkle over a little salt and pepper, and cook until browned, turning frequently.

Reduce the heat to medium-low. Add the onion and cook for 5–6 minutes, until softened, then add the garlic and cook for another minute.

Add the mushrooms and cook for 5–6 minutes, until starting to brown. Add the white wine, then reduce the heat to low and simmer for 40–45 minutes.

Add the crème fraîche and cook for another 10 minutes, then sprinkle over the parsley and serve.

NOTES

Use any combination of chicken you like – we won't judge you.

If freezing, freeze before crème fraiche is added. Defrost thoroughly before cooking.

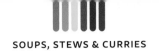

WHAT'S A HOT-POT NOT?

Seriously, readers – on *Strike It Lucky*, when Barrymore used to shout 'What's a hot-spot not' to the audience, what did they shout back? Because hot makes absolutely no sense, and I can't imagine a showman like Barrymore standing for anything other than perfection. Either way, we'll tell you what a hot-pot isn't – quick. But if you persevere with the longer cooking time here, you'll have yourself a meal that will put hairs on your chest.

That analogy doesn't quite work if you're a) wanting to stay clean-shaven, or b) like me, with every square centimetre of skin already growing enough hair out of it to stuff a pillow.

This recipe is adapted from my mother's classic, though I confess we've mixed it up a little by adding flavour. See notes for further thoughts.

SERVES: 4
PREP: 15 minutes
COOK: 1 hour 30 minutes
CALORIES: 383

600g (1lb 5oz) diced beef
1 teaspoon salt
¼ teaspoon black pepper
1 onion, sliced
4 cloves of garlic, crushed
    or grated
1 carrot, peeled and sliced
250ml (9fl oz) beef stock
½ teaspoon thyme
1 tablespoon Worcestershire
    sauce
1 tablespoon tomato purée
3 potatoes
a bunch of fresh parsley, finely
    chopped

Preheat the oven to 180°C fan/400°F/gas mark 6.

Spray an ovenproof pan with a little oil and place over a medium-high heat. Add the beef, sprinkle over the salt and pepper, cook for 5–6 minutes until browned all over, then remove to a plate and keep aside.

Add the onion and cook for 3–4 minutes, until softened. Add the garlic and carrot and stir.

Put the beef back into the pan along with the beef stock, thyme, Worcestershire sauce and tomato purée. Give another good stir, bring to the boil, then remove from the heat.

Thinly slice the potatoes (no need to peel) and place on top of the stew, overlapping them neatly. Spray them with a little oil.

Cover the pan with a lid (or foil) and cook in the oven for 50 minutes.

Remove the lid or foil, increase the temperature to 200°C fan/425°F/gas mark 7, and cook for a further 15 minutes.

Remove from the oven, sprinkle over the parsley, and serve.

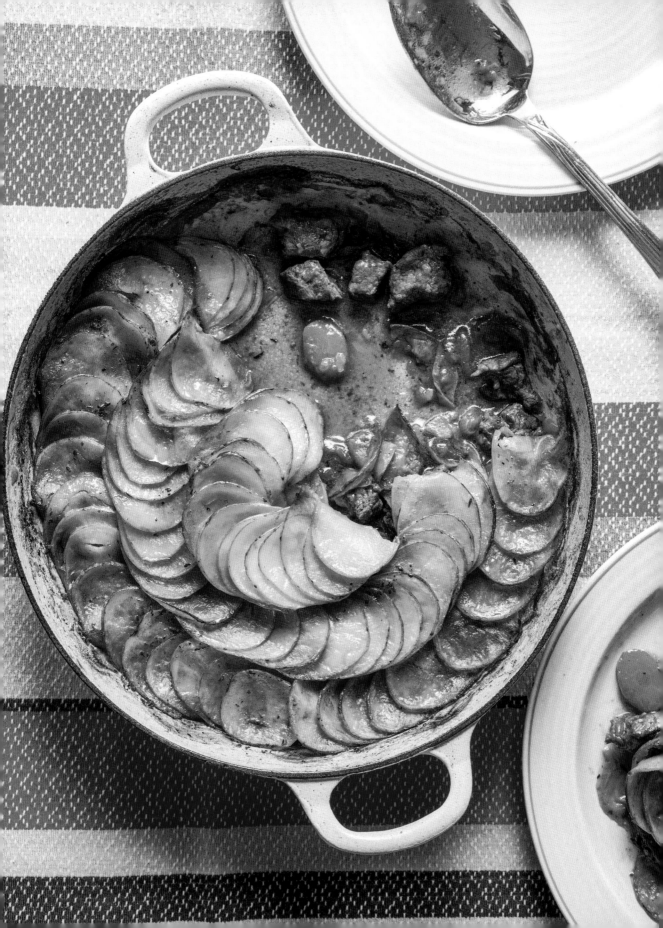

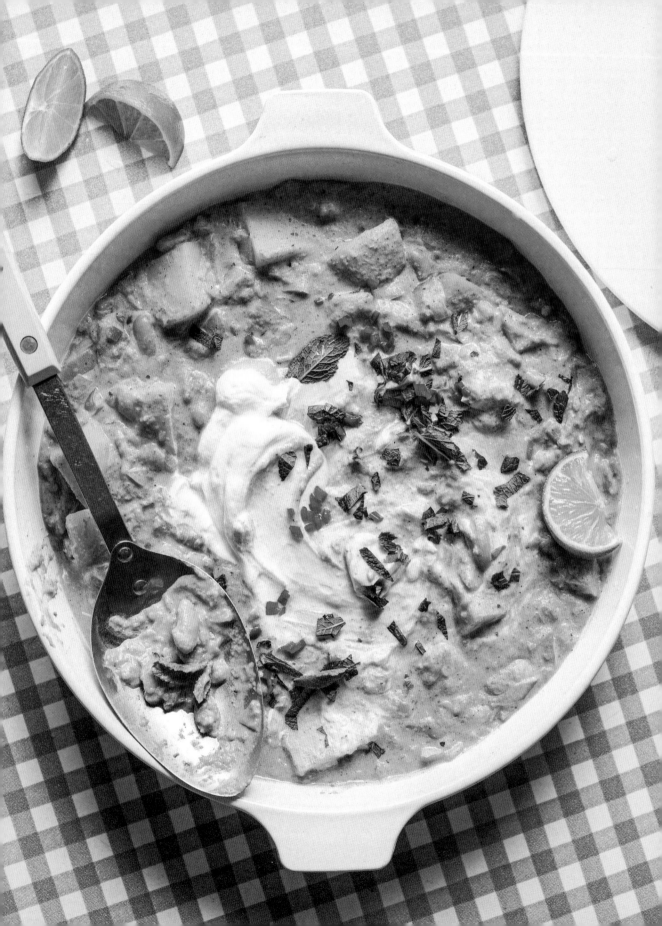

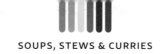
APPLE & CANNELLINI CURRY

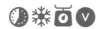

A lickety-split vegetarian curry for your consideration, with the added benefit of some apple, which, if you really think about it, turns this into a dessert. Going without meat for one meal won't kill you off, especially when the dish tastes as good as this.

Mind, this is coming from someone who lives his life constantly thinking he's about to die in some convoluted, start-of-*Casualty* set-up. A good case in point is our garage door – it is ancient old and I once read online that lots of people are killed by the rusty springs tearing free and taking their head clean off. So you can imagine, can't you, my fear and terror every time I need to go into the garage to retrieve something illicit (trade coming over) or hide something illicit (parents coming over)? Luckily, I'm a man who confronts his fears head on, and therefore I bravely elect to send Paul in first. The word hero gets bandied around awful easy these days …

SERVES: 4
PREP: 10 minutes
COOK: 45 minutes
CALORIES: 364

2 large apples, cored
3 potatoes, peeled
3 onions, finely diced
¼ teaspoon salt
1 red chilli, deseeded and
    finely diced
4 cloves of garlic, crushed
2 tablespoons curry powder
500ml (18fl oz) vegetable stock
200g (7oz) tinned cannellini
    beans, drained
150g (5½oz) low-fat soft cheese
1 bunch of fresh mint leaves,
    chopped
200g (7oz) Greek yoghurt
1 lime, quartered

Chop the apples and potatoes into 2cm (¾ inch) cubes (there's no need to peel the apples).

Spray a large saucepan with a little oil and place over a medium heat. Add the onions to the pan along with the salt and cook for about 3–4 minutes, stirring occasionally.

Add the chilli and garlic and cook for a further 2 minutes, then add the curry powder and cook for another 2 minutes.

Add the chopped apples and the vegetable stock, stir well, cover the pan with a lid and cook for 10 minutes.

Carefully spoon out half the curry mix and blend until smooth, then return it to the pan. Add the potatoes, cannellini beans and soft cheese and cook for another 15 minutes, until the potatoes are tender.

Remove from the heat and leave to cool for 5 minutes, then stir in the chopped mint and Greek yoghurt and serve, with lime quarters for squeezing over.

NOTES

Chickpeas work just as well in this – simply swap the same amount for the cannellini beans.

If you're freezing, freeze before stirring in the mint and yoghurt.

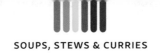

CHICKEN GRAVY CURREH

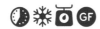

I'm not entirely sure why Paul has spelled curry as curreh, save for the fact that he likes to give our proofreaders something to agonise over while they review our simming (😊) recipes. He does often shout CHICKEN CURREH at me in some weird accent though, so perhaps it is that. Either way, what you have here is a very simple dish which at first glance uses all sorts of spices, but listen, if you haven't got a well-stocked cupboard by now then what's this all been about?

Long-time followers will remember our wonderful spice jars magnetically attached to the side of our fridge, and will doubtless be relieved and able to sleep again to learn they survived the fire.

SERVES: 4
PREP: 15 minutes
COOK: 45 minutes
CALORIES: 295

1 cardamom pod
2 cloves
1 cinnamon stick
1 teaspoon dried chilli flakes
3 onions, finely chopped
2 cloves of garlic, crushed or grated
2½cm (1 inch) piece of root ginger, grated
500g (1lb 2oz) skinless, boneless chicken thighs (or breasts), diced
1 tomato, chopped
2 teaspoons hot chilli powder
3 tablespoons Greek yoghurt
½ teaspoon ground turmeric
½ teaspoon ground coriander
½ teaspoon ground cumin
½ teaspoon garam masala
3 green chillies, sliced
2 tablespoons chopped fresh coriander leaves
½ teaspoon chopped fresh fenugreek leaves
1 tablespoon butter

Spray a large pan with a little oil and place over a medium-high heat. Add the cardamom, cloves, cinnamon and chilli flakes and stir them around the pan.

Add the onions and cook for 4–5 minutes until softened. Add the garlic and ginger and cook for 1 more minute.

Add the chicken to the pan and cook until no pink meat remains. Add the tomato and 1 teaspoon of the hot chilli powder and stir, then cook for 3–4 minutes.

Meanwhile, mix together the yoghurt, the remaining teaspoon of hot chilli powder, the turmeric, ground coriander and cumin in a bowl, and add to the pan along with 125ml (4fl oz) of water. Add the garam masala and cook for a few more minutes.

Stir in the green chillies, coriander leaves and fenugreek leaves and cook for 5 more minutes.

Finally, add the butter and stir until melted through.

Serve with rice.

NOTES

OK, we know there are a lot of ingredients for this, so feel free to swap things out for whatever you have – it'll probably be fine!

Fat-free yoghurt won't work here – it will split. Get the good stuff – you're worth it.

If you haven't got fenugreek leaves you can use ¼ teaspoon of ground fenugreek or mustard seeds instead.

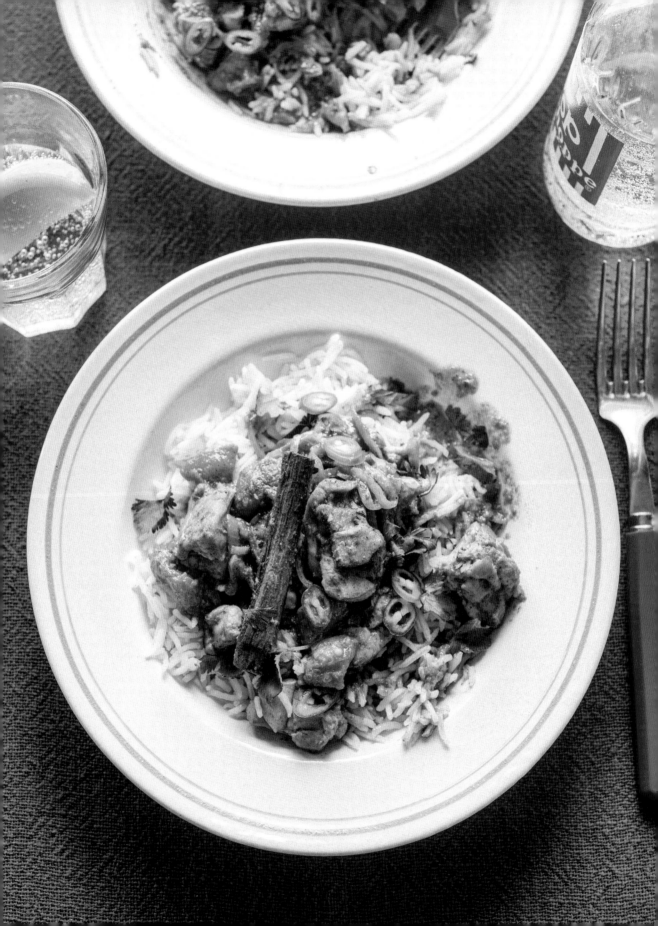

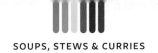
VEGGIE PASANDA

You're right – this is a lot of ingredients, isn't it? But most of them you'll have rattling around in the cupboards and freezer, and those that you don't, you can pick up easily enough. Plus, take a look – a lot of the list is made up from the spice mix we use. I'll keep the recipe intro brief for a change, save to offer up some encouragement: experiment with vegetable curries! There are far better chefs than us out there cooking some delightful, astonishingly good meals with no meat, and there's the added bonus that they'll nearly always be that much cheaper.

SERVES: 4
PREP: 10 minutes
COOK: 25 minutes
CALORIES: 449

3 tablespoons ground almonds
6 carrots, peeled
1 courgette
1 onion, diced
1 cinnamon stick
3 cardamom pods
3 cloves of garlic, crushed
   or grated
1 tablespoon grated ginger
1 teaspoon ground turmeric
1½ teaspoons curry powder
1½ teaspoons ground coriander
¼ teaspoon hot chilli powder
2 tablespoons tomato purée
100g (3½oz) frozen peas
100g (3½oz) mushrooms,
   chopped
1 × 400g (14oz) tin of butter beans
1 vegetable stock cube
4 tablespoons flaked almonds
8 tablespoons Greek yoghurt

Mix the ground almonds with 6 tablespoons of water in a bowl, and set aside.

Trim the carrots and cut into ½cm (¼ inch) slices. Trim the courgette and halve lengthways, then slice into ½cm (¼ inch) half-moon shapes.

Spray a large frying pan with a little oil and place over a medium-high heat. Add the onion, cinnamon and cardamom and cook for 3–4 minutes.

Add the garlic, ginger, turmeric, curry powder, ground coriander and chilli powder and cook for another minute, stirring constantly. Add the tomato purée, ground almond paste and 250ml (9fl oz) of water and stir, then bring to a simmer.

Add the carrots, courgettes, peas, mushrooms and butter beans, crumble in the stock cube, then stir and simmer for 10 minutes. Remove from the heat and set aside to cool for a couple of minutes while you toast the almonds.

Place a small frying pan or saucepan on a low heat, then add the flaked almonds (don't use any oil) and cook for a few minutes, tossing them now and again. Keep an eye on them because they will burn quickly! You're looking for a golden colour. Tip them into a bowl and set aside.

Add the yoghurt to the curry and stir gently.

Top with the toasted almonds and serve with rice.

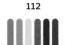

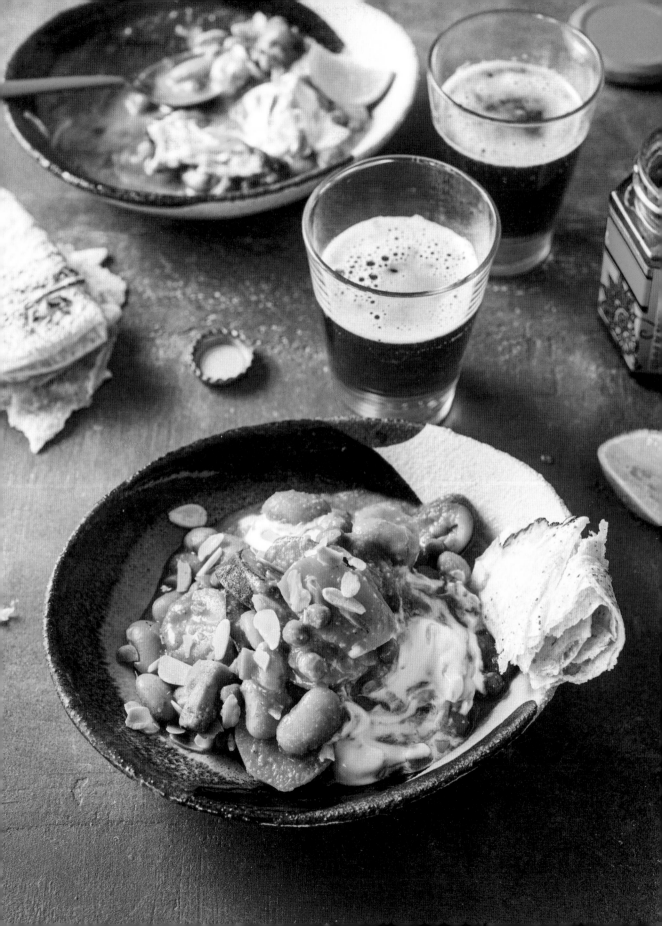

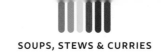
GARLIC CHICKEN CURRY

Between this recipe and the date-wrecking garlic beef in our earlier books, we're on a mission to make sure you stay celibate for the rest of your life. Unless you like the smell of garlic on a lover's breath, in which case, share your dinner, stick a towel down and away you go.

Of course, this only applies if your partner is a good kisser, because frankly there are few things more unattractive than a bad kisser. Back in the days before Paul wandered into my life, I was romantically linked with a lovely chap who had one major flaw: he kissed like Kirby from the old Nintendo games. Google it. A romantic moment should not leave you fearing for your fillings, but no matter how gently I encouraged a more natural approach, he would clamp on to my face and not so much kiss me as hoover my mouth like a car valeter. I broke the relationship off a few weeks later when I realised he was raising the pitch of my voice through kisses alone.

Anyway, moral of the story: if you're planning on necking on, perhaps leave this admittedly delicious dinner for another night, because you'll be absolutely honking of garlic.

SERVES: 4
PREP: 15 minutes
COOK: 30 minutes
MARINATING: 4 hours +
CALORIES: 265

15 cloves of garlic
8 skinless, boneless chicken
   thighs
150g (5½oz) Greek yoghurt
1 teaspoon ground turmeric
2 teaspoons salt
1 green chilli
2cm (¾ inch) piece of ginger,
   thinly sliced
1 red onion, sliced
½ teaspoon sugar
1 teaspoon ground cumin
½ teaspoon ground coriander
½ teaspoon garam masala
½ teaspoon chilli powder
150ml (5fl oz) chicken stock
½ a bunch of fresh coriander,
   roughly chopped

Crush or grate 10 of the garlic cloves into a large bowl. Add the chicken and yoghurt, along with ½ teaspoon of turmeric and 1 teaspoon of salt. Mix gently to ensure the chicken is well coated. Leave to marinate for a minimum of 4 hours, or ideally overnight.

When ready to cook, slice the rest of the garlic and finely chop the green chilli. Spray a large non-stick pan with a little oil and place over a medium heat. Add the garlic and chilli to the pan along with the ginger and cook for a few minutes, until the garlic starts to turn golden.

Add the onion, the rest of the salt and turmeric, the sugar, cumin, ground coriander, garam masala and chilli powder. Stir and cook for 4–5 minutes, until the onion is starting to turn golden.

Add the chicken and its yoghurt marinade to the pan, stir everything well, then cook for 10 minutes, stirring frequently. Add the chicken stock, give another good stir, and cook for a further 10 minutes.

Sprinkle over the coriander and serve.

NOTES

The bigger the garlic cloves, the better.

Don't be tempted to use fat-free yoghurt – it will curdle. Trust us – the good stuff is worth the extra calories.

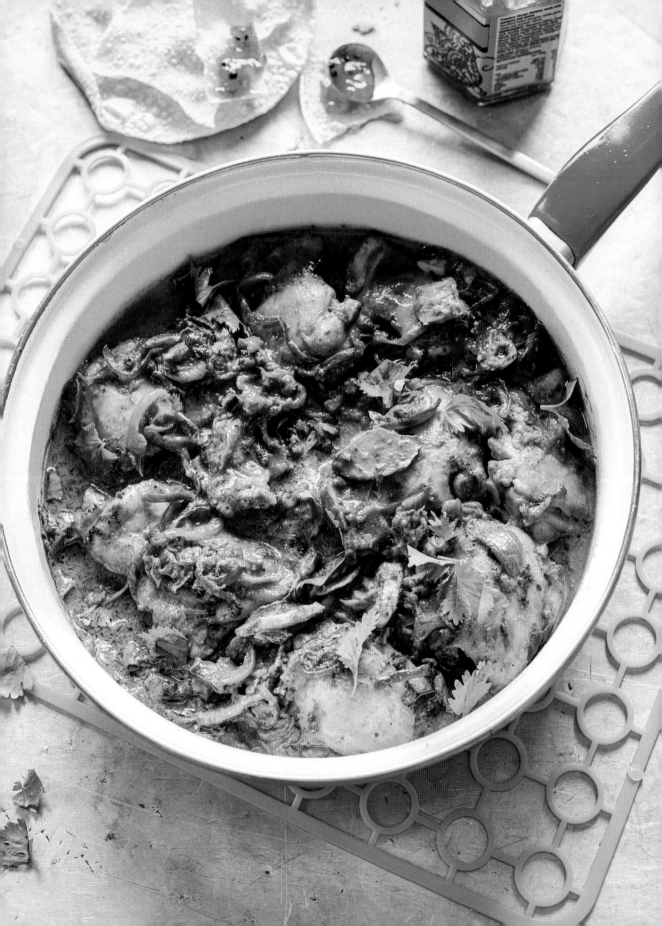

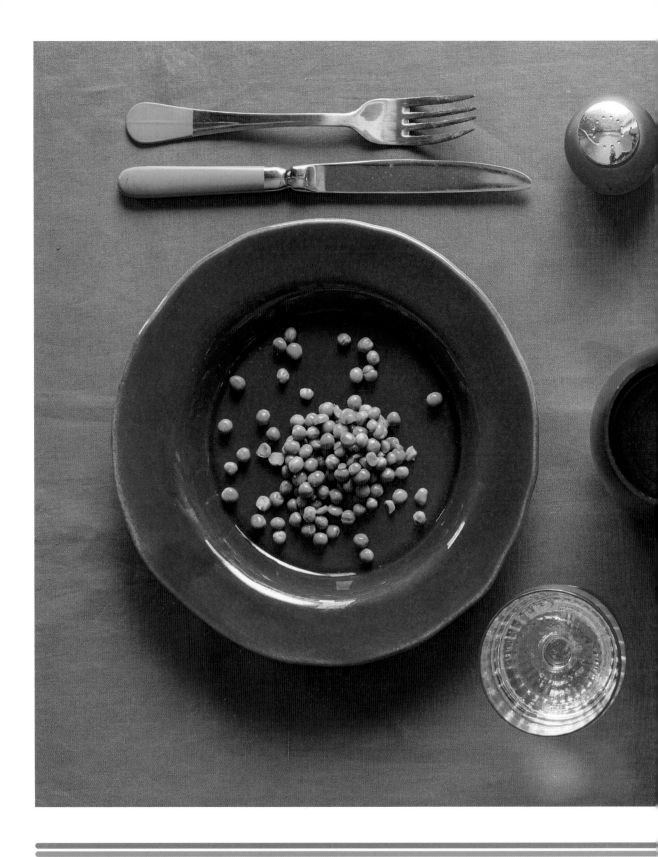

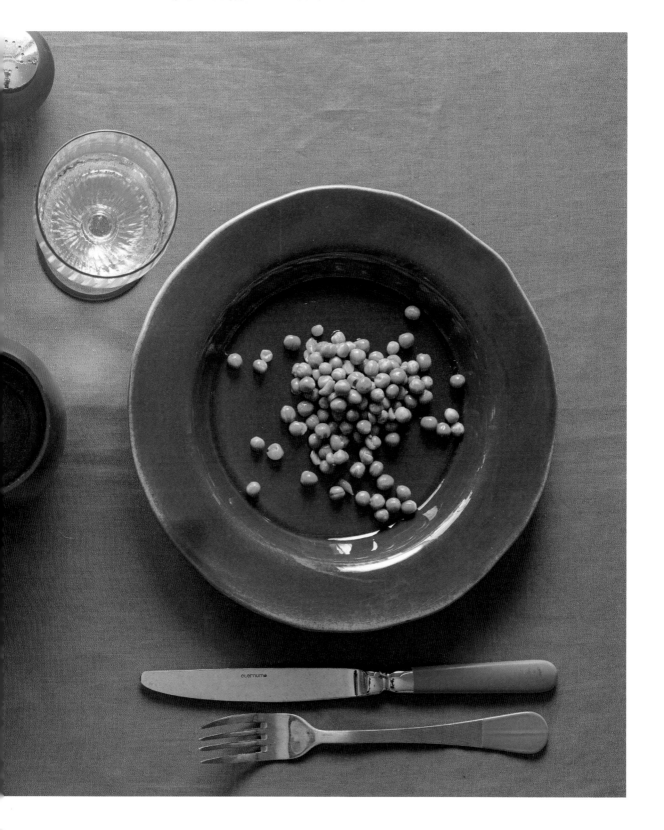

FAST

SEND NOODS LOL

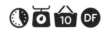

We had a far, far better title for this recipe, but we have sadly/loudly been told it would be ill-advised to use it lest we trigger off someone's sensibilities and get terse direct messages telling us how we should never have been born. So, instead, we've gone for a laboured take on a meme and we hope everyone is as happy as those who live their life to be offended can be. As it happens, we do get a surprising amount of noods sent to us – even more surprising is that it is ladies who insist on sending us them. Don't get us wrong, you're all beautiful, but we aren't suddenly going to forget our homosexual ways.

This meal is a dinner idea, but really one that Paul often takes into work for lunch, given how easily you can take it in a jar and fill it with boiling water when you're ready.

And though this almost goes without saying, you are of course not beholden to the ingredients listed below: you can use any cooked meat or thinly chopped vegetable to make this transportable little dinner your own.

SERVES: 1
PREP: 5 minutes
COOK: 8 minutes
CALORIES: 478

100g (3½oz) dried noodles
30g (1oz) cooked chicken or beef, shredded
½ vegetable stock cube, crumbled
2 teaspoons soy sauce
½ teaspoon sesame oil
2 button mushrooms, thinly sliced
30g (1oz) frozen sweetcorn
25g (1oz) carrot, grated
20g (¾oz) baby spinach, chopped
1 spring onion, thinly sliced

Place all the ingredients together in a jar, pot, bowl or whatever you have to hand.

Pour over 240ml (9fl oz) of boiling water and leave for 6–8 minutes, stirring occasionally.

NOTE

As a fancy bonus, we love soy eggs with these. Simply hard-boil an egg, and while it's cooking mix together 1 crushed clove of garlic, 2 tablespoons of soy sauce, 1 teaspoon of mirin and a pinch of dried chilli flakes. Peel the egg and leave to marinate in the sauce for half an hour.

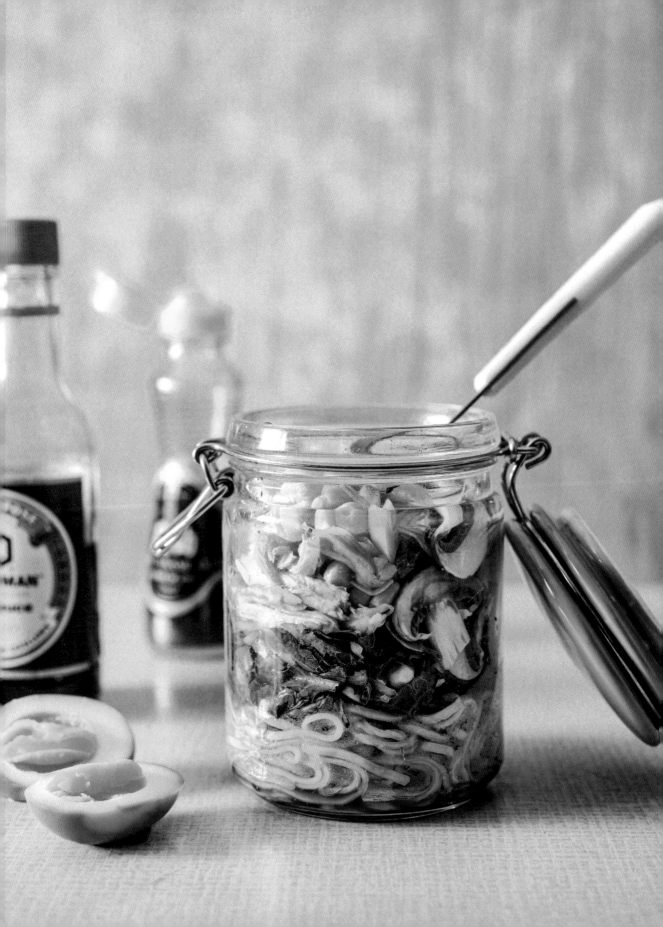

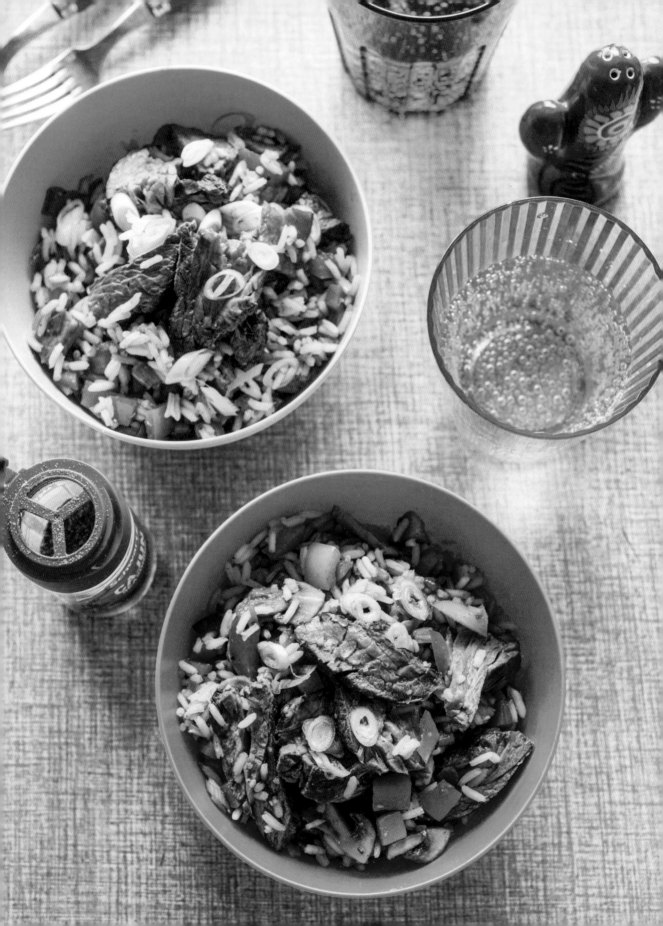

CAJUN STEAK DIRTY RICE

One of our most popular recipes from the blog, although we do hate the title – dirty rice doesn't exactly sound inviting. We apologise for that, but this beefy wonder-dish will liven up any evening plans. You mustn't feel restricted to the vegetables we use – rather like a chow mein, this dish will carry any vegetables you chuck at it, although if we may offer some advice: chop everything finely so it cooks at the same time. Think of this as a more substantial rice salad and you'll be on your way.

SERVES: 4
PREP: 10 minutes
COOK: 20 minutes
CALORIES: 491

250g (9oz) long-grain rice
400g (14oz) steak
4 bacon medallions, diced
½ onion, diced
2 teaspoons Cajun seasoning
1 teaspoon Worcestershire sauce
1 beef stock cube
6 button mushrooms, diced
1 carrot, peeled and finely diced
½ red, ½ yellow and ½ green
    pepper, deseeded and finely
    diced
2 spring onions, finely diced

Cook the rice according to the packet instructions, then drain and set aside.

Spray a large frying pan with a little oil and place over a medium-high heat. Add the steak to the pan and cook to your liking – we like ours medium-rare, so that's about 3–4 minutes each side. The cooking time will depend on the thickness of your steak. Once it's done, remove to a plate and leave to rest.

Wipe out the pan and spray with a little more oil, then put back over the heat. Add the bacon and onion and cook until the bacon is crispy.

Stir in the Cajun seasoning and Worcestershire sauce.

Dissolve the stock cube in 200ml (7fl oz) of boiling water, stir, and keep to one side.

Add the mushrooms, carrots and peppers to the pan along with the stock and give a good stir.

Cook until most of the liquid has evaporated, stirring frequently, then add the rice and mix to warm through.

Dice the steak and add to the pan, stirring once more.

Serve, sprinkled with the spring onions.

NOTES

You don't need fancy or expensive steak for this, any will do.

If you can't be a*sed to cook rice, just use a couple of microwave pouches. Heat in the microwave towards the end of the cooking time and stir into the pan with the vegetables.

The colour of the peppers isn't too important – simply use what you have, it'll still work fine!

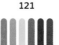

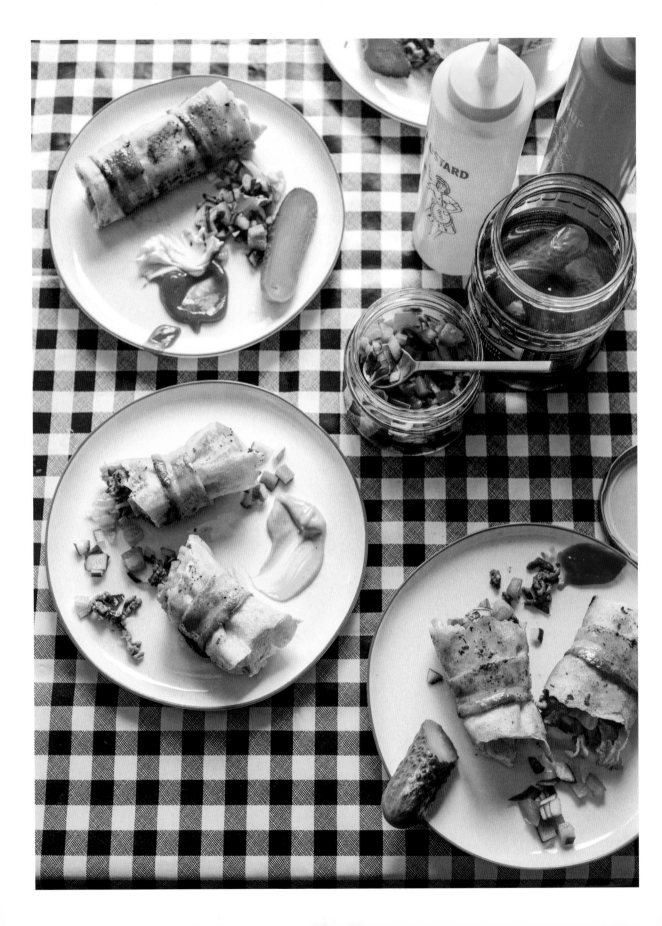

BACON CHEESEBURGER BURRITO

This burrito, stuffed with all the tasty bits of a cheeseburger, came to us via a roadside food truck in Las Vegas, a place where we are almost certainly destined to die in the future. We stopped there for a few days as we minced our way across Canada (we know Las Vegas isn't in Canada, but it's only a short flight and I wanted to gamble some of Paul's pin money away), and boy, was it an assault on the senses. Everything is geared to wonderful excess and we took full advantage, with almost everything that we put in our mouths designed to shorten our life expectancy in delicious, greasy, smoky ways.

We have made a couple of adjustments to bring it more in line with the calories you would expect from us, but for the most part, it remains unchanged. If you wanted to fully replicate our initial experience you would need to drive halfway to the Hoover Dam in a Mustang in which you managed to leave the handbrake on, pull over to investigate the blue smoke and pick up a burrito to calm yourself down. Yes, there were some tense words exchanged that day …

SERVES: 4
PREP: 10 minutes
COOK: 15 minutes
CALORIES: 499

350g (12oz) lean minced beef
4 cloves of garlic, crushed
  or grated
1 tablespoon Worcestershire
  sauce
1 teaspoon black pepper
pinch of salt
2 tablespoons mayonnaise
1 tablespoon tomato ketchup
1 tablespoon mustard
85g (3oz) reduced fat Cheddar
  cheese, grated
4 tortilla wraps
50g (1¾oz) gherkins, finely diced
50g (1¾oz) tomatoes, diced
1 onion, finely diced
60g (2¼oz) iceberg lettuce,
  chopped
8 slices of streaky bacon
salt

Spray a large frying pan with a little oil and place over a medium-high heat. Add the mince, along with the garlic, Worcestershire sauce, pepper and a pinch of salt, cook for 4–5 minutes, until browned, then remove from the heat.

Leave for a few minutes to cool, then stir in the mayonnaise, ketchup and mustard and set aside.

Sprinkle the cheese into the centre of each wrap, then spoon a quarter of the mince mixture into each one.

Top with the gherkins, tomatoes, onion and lettuce, then fold each edge and roll closed to form a burrito. Wrap 2 slices of bacon around each burrito, with the join on the underside.

Wipe the frying pan clean, place back over a medium heat, and spray with a little oil. Cook the burritos for 2–3 minutes each side, until browned and crispy.

Serve!

NOTE

The crispy bacon on the outside really finishes this nicely, but if you're looking to save on some calories you could fry some bacon medallions and wrap them with the mince inside the burrito.

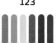

FRITTATA DE CORSE

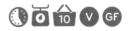

Five ingredients to make an evening meal you can slap together with barely an effort and, when served with beans topped with cheese, will make your belly gurgle with happiness? I know, we are good to you. This brilliantly simple dinner arrives from Corsica, a place where we enjoyed a happy week throwing our mortgage away when we were young and far more flighty. I say young – compared to the people on the plane with us on the flight over we were positively newborn. I'd never seen a stewardess pushing a trolley of Complan and Sanatogen down the aisle before. I mean, Paul and I aren't exactly ones for a hedonistic lifestyle, but I've never felt like such a go-getter, clattering down those aeroplane steps at Figari airport and being the only one who wasn't being led down by their elbow. Honestly, it was like the world's slowest conga-line.

Corsica is also where I first learned Paul could sail a boat – not because we went out on the sea, hell no, I barely trust Paul to direct me in bed, let alone on water – but simply because every time we passed a beautiful yacht he would turn to me and mention he was a fully trained sailor. He does the same whenever Warwick Davies is on the telly, lest I've somehow forgotten in the week and a half since he last told me that they grew up in the same village together. Frankly, I don't understand how Paul could have a childhood that encompassed learning to sail but somehow missed out being able to eat without cascading two-thirds of what is meant for his mouth all down the front of his shirt.

SERVES: 4
PREP: 10 minutes
COOK: 15 minutes
CALORIES: 298

500g (1lb 2oz) potatoes
6 eggs
1 tablespoon dried herbes
   de Provence
120g (4½oz) soft goat's cheese
1 bunch of mint leaves, roughly
   chopped

Peel the potatoes and chop into 2cm (¾ inch) cubes, then put them into a large saucepan of boiling water. Cook for 5 minutes, until tender, then drain.

Crack the eggs into a bowl and beat with the herbes de Provence. Stir in the potatoes.

Spray a large frying pan with a little oil and place over a medium-high heat.

Pour the egg mix into the pan, crumble in the goat's cheese, and sprinkle in the mint. When the edges are set but the middle is still a little bit runny, turn out on to a plate.

Cut into wedges and serve.

NOTE

Goat's cheese isn't for everyone, we know. Soft cheese will also do the trick.

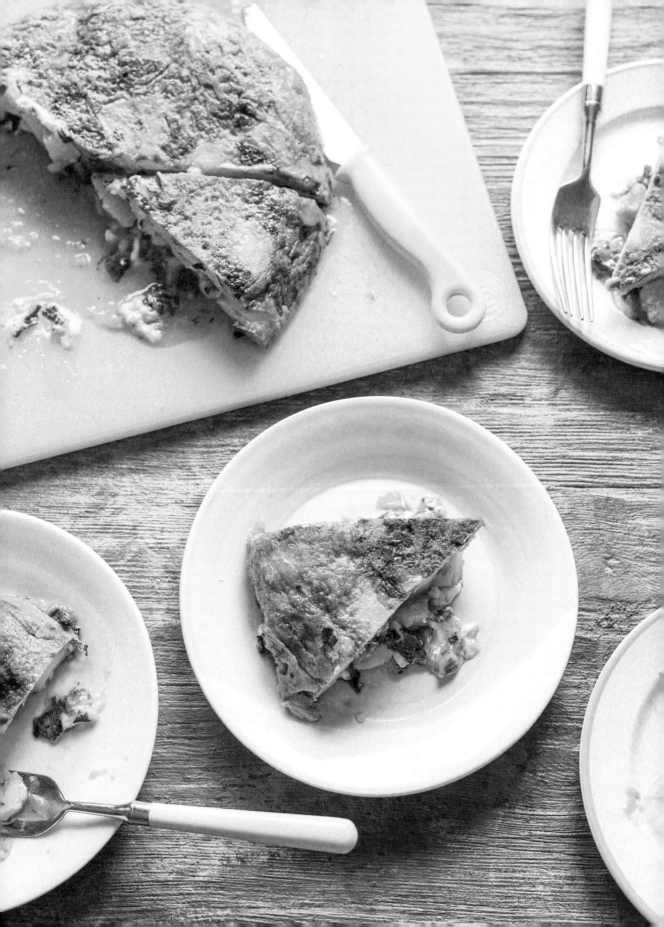

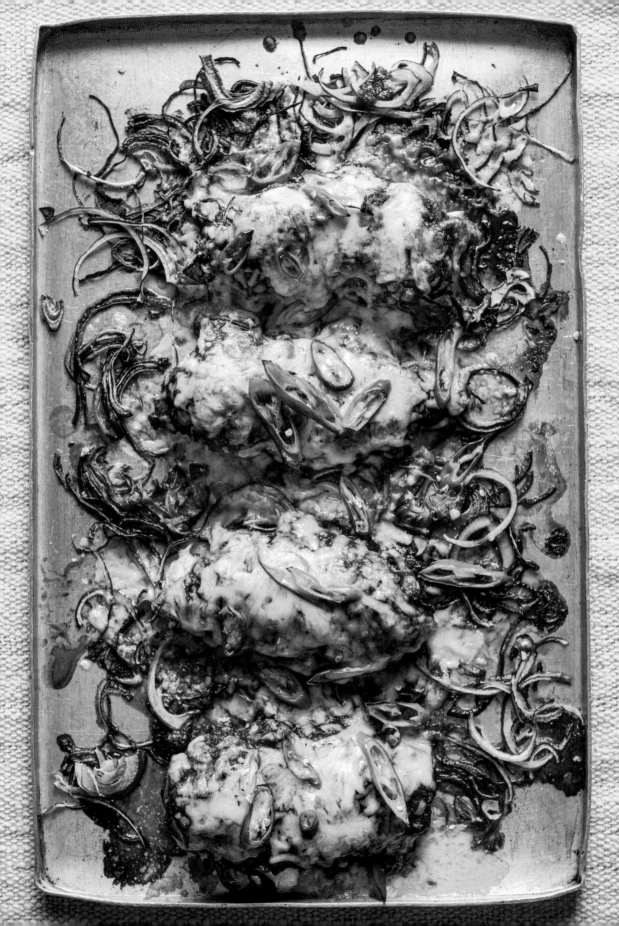

FOXY HUNTER'S CHICKEN

Ah, Hunter's Chicken: the recipe du jour of every slimming soul for a good few months. It's understandable why – anything that combines cheese, spicy sauce and chicken is always going to be a winner. The dish does rather put me in mind of those terrible chain restaurants attached to roadside hotels, where the chicken has been cooked four days before you arrive and the sauce is a gelatinous ode to disappointment. Not here, we promise: this is a dish for the ages.

I say that with utter hypocrisy, mind: I bloody love those places. As long as you're comfortable with high levels of stodge and low levels of flavour, they're a winner. Plus let's be fair, I do some of my best work in those roadside hotels …

SERVES: 4
PREP: 10 minutes
COOK: 25 minutes
CALORIES: 479

4 skinless, boneless chicken
   breasts
8 rashers of streaky bacon
2 red onions, sliced
100g (3½oz) barbecue sauce
2 tablespoons tomato sauce
1 tablespoon sriracha
2 teaspoons Worcestershire
   sauce
1 teaspoon onion granules
1 teaspoon garlic granules
2 teaspoons smoked paprika
50g (1¾oz) mozzarella cheese,
   grated
50g (1¾oz) reduced-fat Cheddar
   cheese, grated
2 green chillies, sliced

Preheat the oven to 200°C fan/425°F/gas mark 7.

Wrap each chicken breast with 2 rashers of bacon and place on a baking sheet, then toss over the sliced onions.

Bake in the oven for 20–25 minutes.

Meanwhile, mix together the barbecue, tomato, sriracha and Worcestershire sauces, along with the onion and garlic granules, and the paprika.

Remove the chicken from the oven and smother with the sauce, then sprinkle over the cheeses and top with the sliced chillies.

Return to the oven, cook for 2 more minutes until the cheese has melted, then serve.

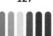

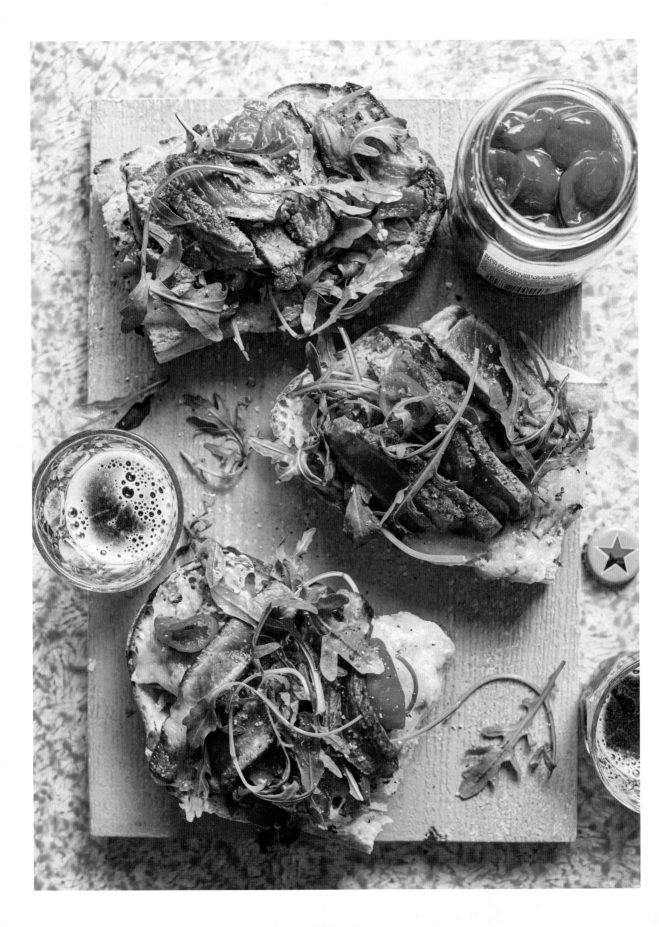

THE BEST STEAK OPEN SANDWICH EVER
AND I WON'T HAVE ANYONE TELL ME OTHERWISE

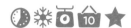

We always go back and forth on the idea of including sandwiches in our books, because honestly, what are they if not just bread with meat stuffed in? But the irrefutable fact is that SANDWICHES ARE THE BEST THING IN THE WORLD. The best part of any funeral, aside from watching long-estranged drunk family members bitch at one another, is the buffet sandwiches at the wake. Meetings at work are more tolerable with sandwich catering. Husband left you for some fancy-piece from the office? Have a delicious sandwich and the world seems that bit brighter, no?

In fact, if I were to marry again, the ideal wedding reception would be with trestle tables adorned with sandwiches, baps, subs and stotties of every filling. At the end of the night I'd explain to Paul that I was far too full for any midnight-malarkey, and that we would take care of things in the morning. A boy can dream. Meanwhile, you must try this steak sandwich, as it is the best we have ever done and Paul will cry if you refuse.

SERVES: 4
PREP: 10 minutes
COOK: 25 minutes
CALORIES: 498

2 ciabattas
2 tablespoons butter
6 cloves of garlic, crushed
   or grated
15g (½oz) fresh parsley, finely
   chopped
4 slices of Manchego cheese
   (80g/2¾oz)
2 steaks
4 handfuls of rocket leaves
12 sweet piquante peppers

NOTES

We're big fans of Manchego, but if you can't get it easily, any cheese will do. Edam and Emmental are great alternatives, and Cheddar also works really well. Use what you have!

This is great as a lunch or brunch, and even better with chips and a side salad (if you're feeling fancy).

Preheat the oven to 200°C fan/425°F/gas mark 7.

Slice the ciabattas in half horizontally and set aside.

Place a small saucepan on a low heat, then add the butter and stir until melted. Add the garlic and parsley, stir, and cook for 3 minutes. Remove from the heat and spoon or brush the butter over the cut sides of the ciabattas. Pop the two slices of ciabatta back together, wrap in foil, and bake in the oven for 10 minutes.

Remove the ciabattas from the oven and set the grill to high. Unwrap the ciabattas and slice in half widthways, then across to give a total of 8 square-ish slices for 4 sandwiches. Top with the slices of cheese and cook under the grill for 3–4 minutes, until the cheese has melted, then set aside.

Spray a frying pan with a little oil and place over a high heat. Add the steaks to the pan and cook for 2–3 minutes each side (or to your liking), then remove to a chopping board. Leave to rest for a few minutes, then slice.

Divide the steak, rocket and peppers between 4 of the ciabatta slices, sandwich with the other 4, and serve.

HALLOUMI WRAPS

The last time we included halloumi in a recipe, we used the entire opening paragraph to squeeze in as many cheese puns as I could possibly manage. To repeat the joke would be both infantile and derivative, and anyway, out of respect for the victims of the Fauxtown Cheese Factory Explosion in 2020, let's keep things respectful.

These halloumi wraps really are something quite terrific, and all the little extras play a part. Go all out and make sure you include everything we mention below. Plus, as an extra tip: sweet chilli sauce drizzled all over your wrap will ensure you have a wonderful time.

SERVES: 4
PREP: 10 minutes
COOK: 15 minutes
CALORIES: 473

2 tablespoons balsamic vinegar
2 teaspoons brown sugar
1 aubergine, sliced
¼ teaspoon salt
¼ teaspoon pepper
1 teaspoon dried oregano
220g (8oz) halloumi cheese, cut into fingers
2 teaspoons capers
120g (4¼oz) sun-dried tomatoes, drained and finely chopped
4 tortillas
4 handfuls of rocket leaves
1 red onion, peeled and sliced

For the tzatziki
½ cucumber, deseeded and grated
6 tablespoons fat-free Greek yoghurt
½ teaspoon garlic granules
½ teaspoon dried dill
½ teaspoon black pepper
½ teaspoon salt

Preheat the oven to 180°C fan/400°F/gas mark 6.

Mix together the tzatziki ingredients and set aside.

Mix the balsamic vinegar and brown sugar in a large bowl, then add the sliced aubergine, salt, pepper and oregano and toss to combine.

Line a baking sheet with greaseproof paper. Add the slices of aubergine in a single layer, and spray with a little oil.

Scatter the halloumi among the aubergine, and bake in the oven for 10–12 minutes.

Meanwhile, mash the capers with the back of a fork and mix with the sun-dried tomatoes.

Spread the mix over one side of the tortillas and top with the rocket leaves.

Add the halloumi and roasted aubergine, drizzle with the tzatziki and sprinkle over the sliced onions.

Tuck and wrap the tortillas, and serve.

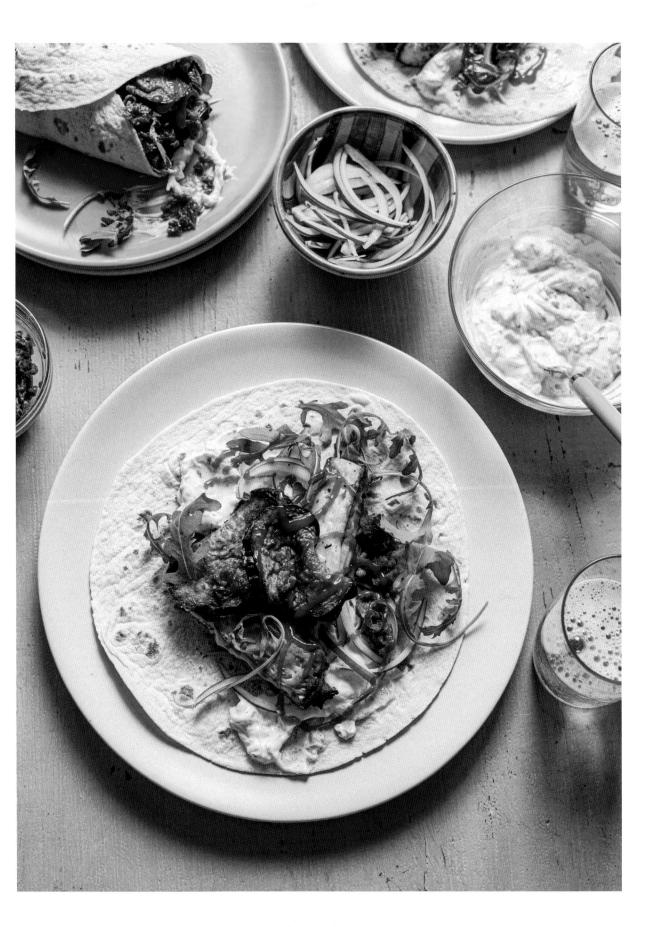

THE GRAND MACKENZIE NOT-TACO TACOS

Wondering about the title? But of course you are. See, Paul calls this meal by another name, and while any budding cruciverbalists among you may be able to work out the original title from the cryptic version above, we don't want the angry clown after us for trademark infringement. Plus, Paul also calls these tacos, which they're absolutely not, but we have to indulge him sometimes. Next he'll be calling hamburgers steamed hams (despite the fact they're obviously grilled).

Speaking of trademarks, one of the most wonderful parts about twochubbycubs finally gaining traction was being able to give up my day job as a trademark legal-person and become a full-time author. If you'll forgive me an indulgence here, I ought to thank you all for making that happen – it's a genuine life goal ticked off. Paul continues to work because he's very important and busy, of course, but I do feel one step closer to having a cottage by a lake where I can smoke a pipe and write and look wistfully out of the window with a hot cup of tea clasped in both hands.

Though, knowing our luck, it'll go all Misery within a week. Which is a shame because I bloody love my left foot.

SERVES: 4
PREP: 5 minutes
COOK: 10 minutes
CALORIES: 500

400g (14oz) lean beef mince
1 onion, finely diced
4 tablespoons reduced-fat
    Thousand Island dressing
4 sesame seed buns, sliced in half
16 sliced gherkins (or as many
    as you like)
½ an iceberg lettuce, sliced
75g (2½oz) Cheddar cheese,
    grated

NOTE

If you're wondering why we simmer the onions – it helps to take the 'sting' out and make them more burger-ish. By all means, though, have them raw if you prefer!

Spray a large frying pan with a little oil and place over a medium-high heat. Add the mince and cook for a few minutes, until browned.

Meanwhile, bring a small saucepan of water to the boil and add the onions. Simmer for 30 seconds, then drain in a sieve and set aside.

While the mince is still cooking, divide the dressing between the bun halves and spread.

Add a couple of slices of gherkins to each bun half and sprinkle over the lettuce and diced onion.

When the mince has finished cooking, spoon on to the bun halves and sprinkle over the cheese.

Fold in half, and enjoy!

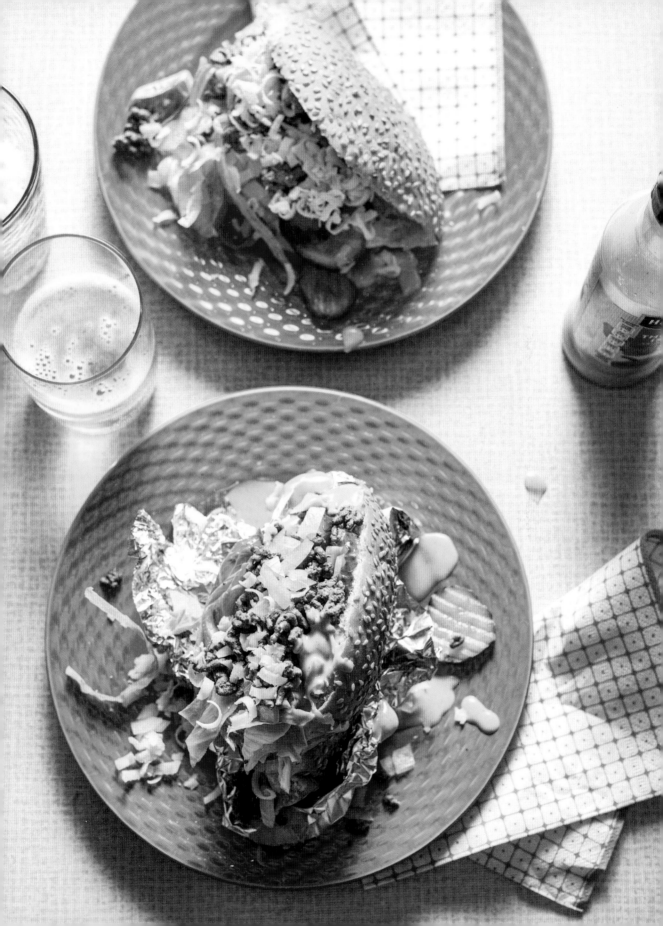

FOREST COUSCOUS

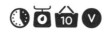

You must understand we're calling this forest couscous because it has mushrooms and garlic in it, which both grow in forests. It's really that simple and I should not have to explain these things to you by now. We know that mushrooms aren't for everyone – to me (James, the one with taste) they're delicious and meaty, whereas Paul (the one with the tastebuds you might expect a long-deceased corpse to share) thinks they're squeaky balls of poison. Clearly he's wrong, but if you are of a similar predisposition, please give a few varieties a go before you condemn them for ever. That's the thing with fungi – they'll grow on you.

Please, though, I beg of you once more: don't be off gallivanting in the forest looking for mushrooms to try and save a few bob. The very last thing Chubby Towers needs is an inquest as to why Sandra from Basingstoke died of fright at the sight of a rainbow-breathing dragon emerging from her oven like that time Bobby from *Home & Away* came out of the fridge to scare Ailsa.

SERVES: 4
PREP: 10 minutes
COOK: 10 minutes
CALORIES: 248

30g (1oz) salted butter
250g (9oz) fancy mushrooms, roughly chopped
5 cloves of garlic, crushed or grated
½ teaspoon dried thyme
150g (5½oz) couscous (plain, but if you're really a fan of the mushroom, use mushroom couscous!)
200ml (7fl oz) vegetable stock
2 tablespoons grated Parmesan or vegetarian Italian-style hard cheese
a pinch of salt and black pepper

On a low heat, gently melt the butter in a frying pan and add the mushrooms and garlic, cooking them slowly to soften, adding the thyme after a minute or two.

Put the couscous into a bowl and cover with the stock, then stir through the butter, mushrooms and garlic, cover with a tight-fitting lid, and leave for about 5 minutes.

Fluff with a fork, season with salt and pepper, and serve topped with the Parmesan.

NOTES

When we say fancy mushrooms, we mean those packs in Tesco that have a good mixture of different fungi in them, but don't stress if you're a button mushroom sort of person – use those instead.

You're right – that is a lot of garlic. But trust us!

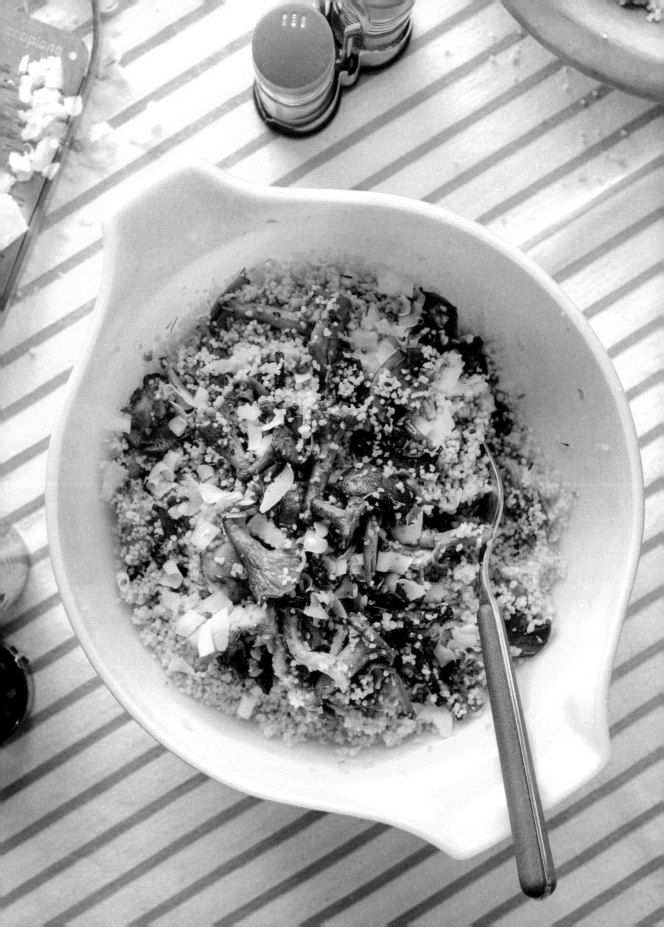

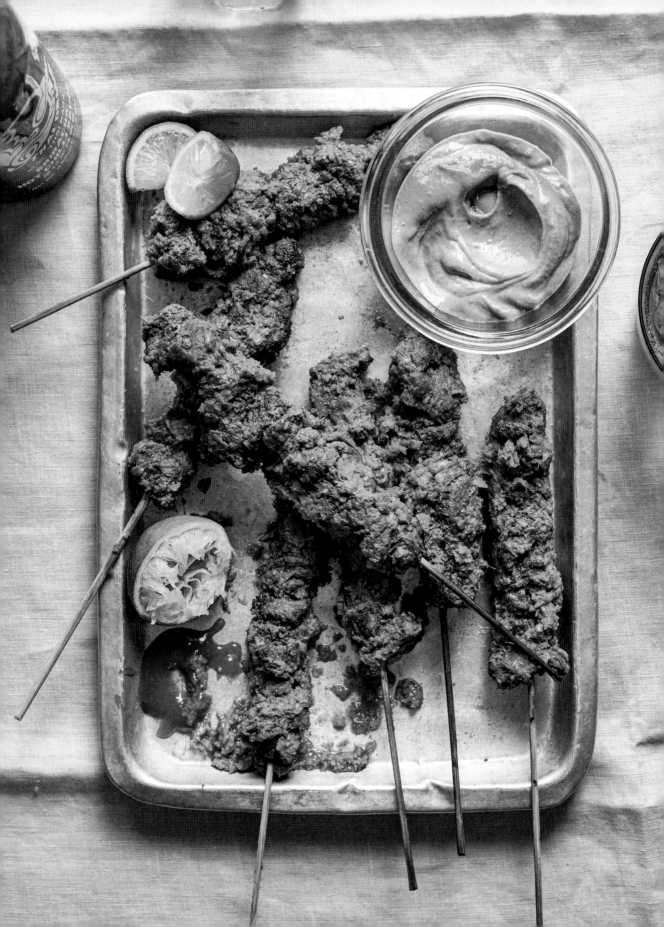

BEEF SATAY WITH DIPPING SAUCE

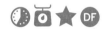

If you were to ask us which of the recipes from the blog we could cheerfully eat all day long and for time evermore, it would be this one. There's something about the dipping sauce – so easy and uncluttered in its simplicity – that I would cheerfully take a bath in. If you're not a fan of peanut butter, then I am afraid we can do nothing for you here, though if it is a dislike borne of breakfasts involving that sugary sweet, claggy paste that came in the pot with the yellow lid, then we urge you to try it again with a decent version.

Though we have suggested you skewer the beef here, there's absolutely nothing stopping you taking it off the skewers after cooking and having yourself a little beefy fondue moment instead. You do you, my love, as no one does it better.

SERVES: 4
PREP: 15 minutes
COOK: 15 minutes
MARINATING: 6 hours +
CALORIES: 381

8 shallots, or 2 onions
2½cm (1 inch) piece of ginger, grated
2 lemongrass stalks
1½ teaspoons ground coriander
1½ teaspoons ground turmeric
1 teaspoon ground cumin
1 teaspoon ground fennel seed
1 teaspoon salt
700g (1lb 9oz) diced beef
1 lime, quartered

For the dipping sauce
4 tablespoons reduced-fat peanut butter
2 tablespoons soy sauce
2 drops of sriracha
1 clove of garlic, crushed or grated

Put all the ingredients (except the beef, and the sauce stuff) into a food processor and pulse until you have a thick paste. Loosen with a few tablespoons of water if it's too thick.

In a large bowl, mix the paste with the beef until well coated, then leave to marinate for at least 6 hours, or ideally overnight.

Thread the beef on to skewers and grill under a high heat for 15 minutes, turning regularly.

Meanwhile, mix together all the dipping sauce ingredients and set aside.

Serve the beef with the sauce on the side and lime quarters for squeezing over.

NOTE

Perfect served with any of our 5 ways sides across the book (minus the soups).

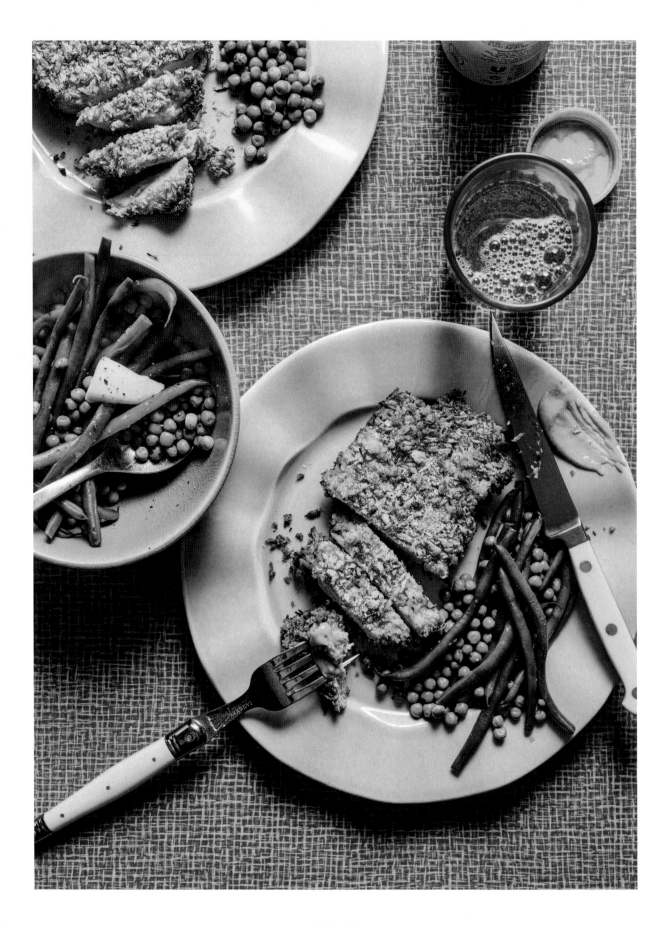

SCHNITZEL

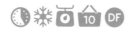

Another thing we brought back from our weekends in Germany – and perhaps the only thing that can't be treated with a course of strong antibiotics – the schnitzel. We have wanted to do one of these for a couple of years now, but it's very much a 'holiday' food for us, in that we don't like to eat it at home because it triggers off our wanderlust and, well, 2020 wasn't exactly the time to be cutting about the globe on a whim.

However, we perfected it during those many weeks in lockdown and can now give you what will doubtless be the most inauthentic – but healthy – take on it.

Oh, and we know schnitzel is technically an Austrian dish, but we've only ever gobbled it in Germany, so hush that voice of dissent.

SERVES: 4
PREP: 10 minutes
COOK: 15 minutes
CALORIES: 470

4 pork loin steaks, all visible
    fat removed
120g (4½oz) panko breadcrumbs
zest of 1 lemon
1 teaspoon dried oregano
1 teaspoon dried thyme
1 tablespoon paprika
2 eggs
2 tablespoons plain flour

Preheat the oven to 200°C fan/425°F/gas mark 7.

Wrap each pork steak loosely in clingfilm and bash with a rolling pin or the bottom of a heavy saucepan until about 1cm (½ inch) thick.

In a shallow dish mix together the panko breadcrumbs, lemon zest, oregano, thyme and paprika. Beat the egg and place in another shallow dish. Put the flour into a third dish.

Gently dredge each of the pork steaks in the flour, then dip in the egg and coat with the breadcrumbs.

Put the steaks on a non-stick baking tray, spray with a little oil and bake in the oven for about 15 minutes.

NOTES

Serve this with whatever you like! We usually have chips and peas because we're rough, but it's also nice with a decent potato salad or some greens.

If freezing, do so before cooking but make sure you defrost thoroughly before cooking.

PITTAWURST

You will spot a couple of German recipes in this book and for that we make no apologies: if we could move to Germany tomorrow, and that supposes that somehow Canada and its lands of bearded wonders and poutine have fallen off the map, then we would. There's something so appealing about a country that seems to run so efficiently, whether it's the public transport system or the fabulous array of sandwiches you see on every corner. Plus, on an entirely shallow note, the fact that almost every word spoken in a male German voice sounds slightly authoritative would leave us permanently excited.

We are yet to have a bad holiday in Germany, even if we do always return to the UK with our belts slightly extended and our feet swollen. We can't help but feel our love is only ever bolstered by the fabulous snacks and takeaways, and these pittawurst sandwiches are an excellent, delicious example of that.

SERVES: 4
PREP: 5 minutes
COOK: 25 minutes
CALORIES: 324

1 onion, sliced
1 green pepper, deseeded and
    sliced
4 bratwurst sausages
60g (2¼oz) reduced-fat crème
    fraîche
1 tablespoon wholegrain mustard
4 wholemeal pitta breads
120g (4½oz) sauerkraut

Preheat the grill to medium-high.

Spray a saucepan with a little oil and place over a medium heat. Add the sliced onion and green pepper and cook for 15 minutes, until softened, stirring occasionally.

Meanwhile, place the bratwursts under the grill and cook for 8–10 minutes, turning frequently. Remove from the grill and slice.

In a small bowl, mix together the crème fraîche and mustard.

Put the pitta breads into a microwave and cook for 15–30 seconds, until they puff up, then remove.

Slice each pitta in half widthways to give 8 'pockets'. Spread the crème fraîche and mustard mix inside, then spoon in the sauerkraut, the onion and pepper mix, and finally stuff with the sliced sausages.

NOTE
We used bratwursts for this, but really any sausage will do!

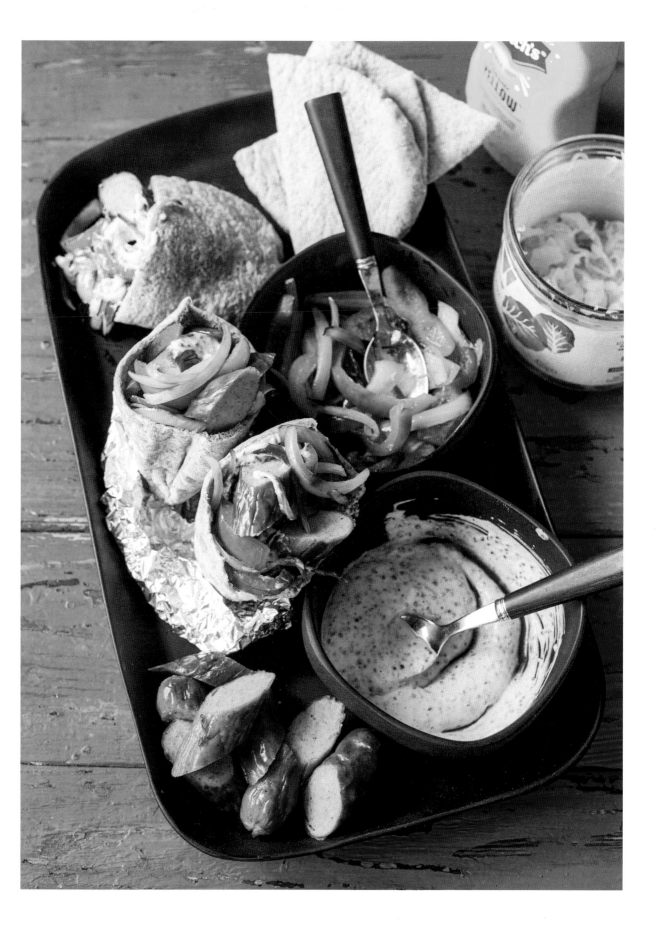

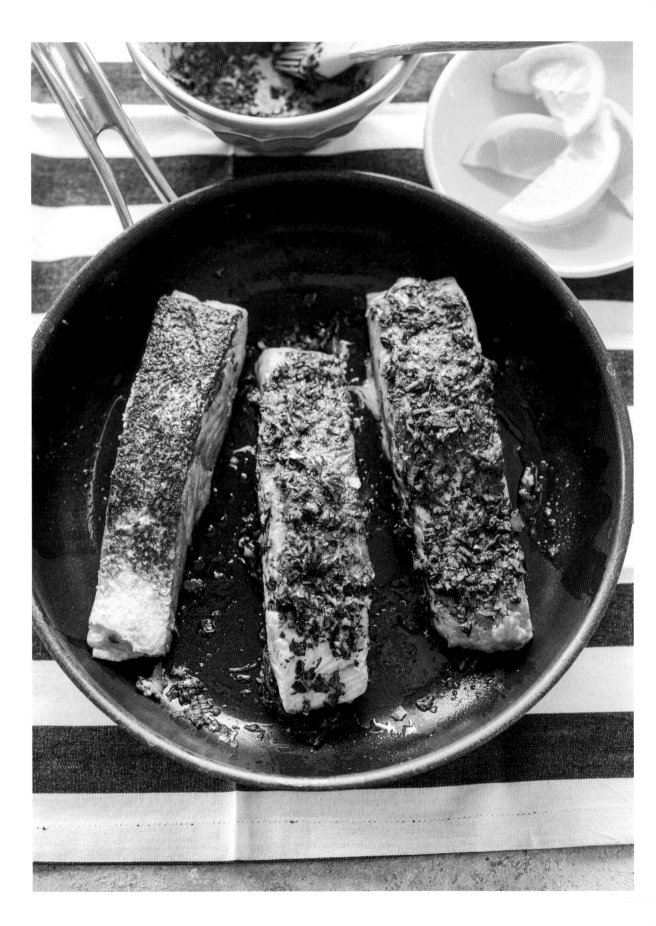

SALMON A LA PLANCHA

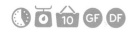

Salmon – the one fish that continues to make an absolute mockery of our oft-repeated claim that we dislike seafood. But what's one more paradox? You can keep those skin-shaving pieces of salmon that fussy people top bagels with, and the less said about salmon roe the better, but a good piece of salmon, cooked perfectly with just a few other ingredients to adorn it, works ever so well.

Mind, salmon also plays havoc with our natural propensity towards procrastination. We buy lots of food with the good intention of cooking it that night, but when the dark draws in, we'll often postpone cooking a new meal, and instead rustle up something simple or from the freezer of mystery. You can't do that with salmon: leave it for more than a moment and it goes all slimy and terrible and fit only for giving to our cats. Happily, this recipe takes mere minutes and requires nothing more than a bit of fussing with a frying pan and making a nice salad to go on the side.

I'm forever leaving projects half-done and coming back to them later, when they make no sense: it's a genuine character flaw. Yet I've tried everything to get past my procrastination, including … (we dare you to find the rest of this sentence later in the book!).

SERVES: 4
PREP: 5 minutes
COOK: 8 minutes
CALORIES: 390

2 cloves of garlic, crushed
    or grated
3 tablespoons finely chopped
    fresh parsley
zest of 1 lemon
2 tablespoons olive oil
4 skin-on salmon fillets
½ teaspoon black pepper
½ teaspoon salt

Mix together the garlic, parsley and lemon zest with 1 tablespoon of the olive oil and set aside.

Brush the salmon on both sides with the remaining tablespoon of olive oil and sprinkle with the salt and pepper.

Spray a large frying pan with a little oil and place over a medium-high heat. Place the salmon in the pan, skin side down, and cook for 4 minutes, then gently turn and cook for 3–4 minutes on the other side.

Remove from the pan and serve skin side up.

Gently spread the garlic mix over the top of the salmon and serve.

OUR OWN COMFORT BOWL CHOICES

We couldn't do a recipe book of evening meals without including the two evening meals we always turn to when we just can't be a*sed. We can't pretend there's any skill or beauty to either of these meals. But sometimes you just want some sheer bloody stodge and there's no shame in that.

PAUL'S 'THINKS HE'S SOMETHING SPECIAL' DINNER

SERVES: 2
PREP: 5 minutes
COOK: 10 minutes
CALORIES: 498

2 hard-boiled eggs
1 tin of tuna
enough salad cream to comfortably drown a Shetland pony
300g (10½oz) cooked pasta
black pepper

Mash the eggs and tuna with the salad cream.

Stir through the pasta.

Heat in the microwave and cover with black pepper.

Sit and eat your dinner, wondering why your partner never kisses you intimately any more.

JAMES'S HOT-DOG DIP

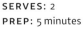

SERVES: 2
PREP: 5 minutes
COOK: 10 minutes
CALORIES: 427

1 tin of hot dogs
2 tins of baked beans
3 large eggs
1 tablespoon chilli sauce

Chop the hot dogs into bits and stir them through the beans.

Slop into a small Pyrex dish and create wells for the eggs.

Crack the eggs into the wells and cover with beans as best you can.

Drizzle chilli sauce on top and cook in the oven on 180°C/400°F/gas mark 6 until the whites of the eggs are just set.

Eat it straight out of the dish while shouting at the telly.

NOTE

Paul sometimes thins the salad cream out with more vinegar because he likes to feel alive once in a while.

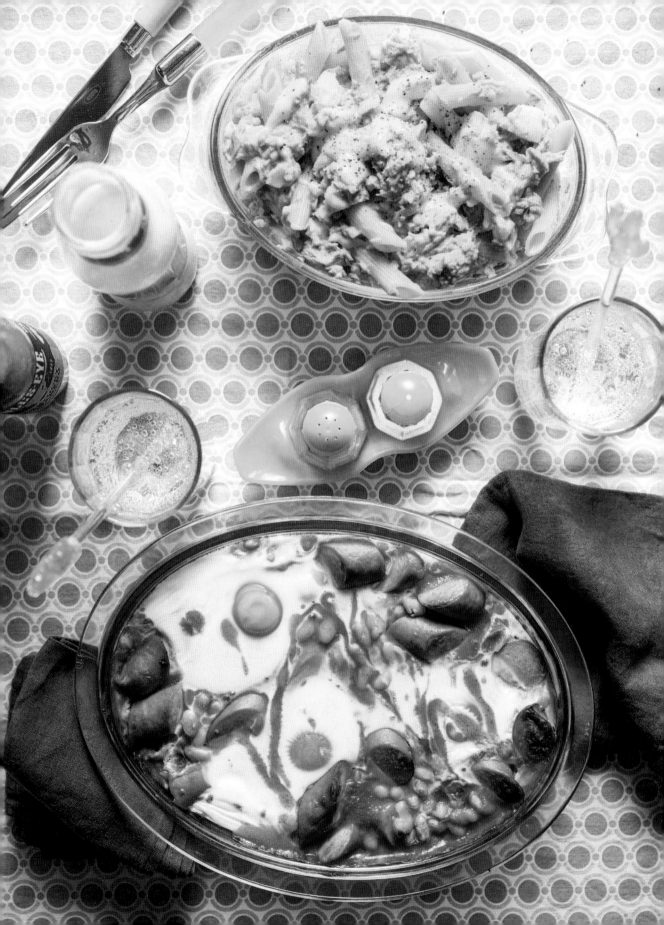

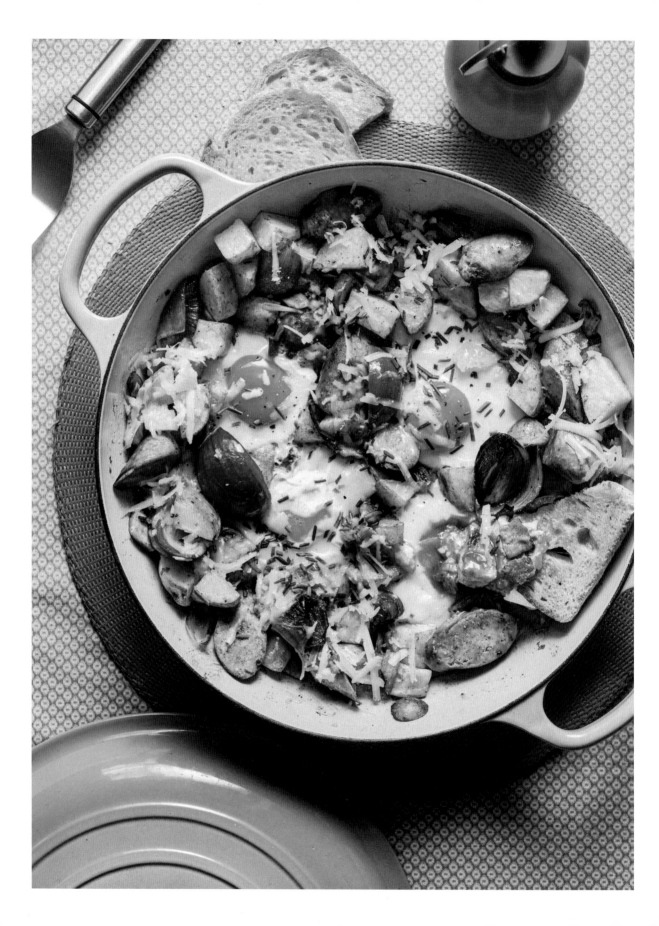

HASH FOR DAYS

We're not sure this is technically a hash, but humour us: it has all the wonderful things of a good breakfast but boosted for some evening sustenance. Slathered with brown sauce (or ketchup, if you're a pervert), this is a dinner that'll use up your bits and bobs from the fridge and leave you with a smile on your face.

You'll note we reference an air-fryer – our favourite piece of kitchen kit. If you're pushed for time, you could absolutely throw the sausages in with the potatoes to cook alongside, then add the bacon and onion when there's about ten minutes to go. Once done, take the paddle out (if your model has one) and crack the eggs straight in. Saves on the washing-up!

SERVES: 4
PREP: 10 minutes
COOK: 25 minutes
CALORIES: 434

4 potatoes
4 low-fat sausages
1 red onion, peeled and quartered
4 bacon medallions
40g (1½oz) button mushrooms, sliced
4 eggs
60g (2¼oz) reduced-fat Cheddar cheese, grated
½ teaspoon chives, sliced

Roughly dice the potatoes into 2cm (¾ inch) chunks (no need to peel) and parboil for 5 minutes, then drain.

Rough up the potatoes in a pan, then either tip into an air-fryer with a drizzle of oil, or roast in the oven for 30 minutes at 200°C fan/425°F/ gas mark 7.

Meanwhile, spray a large frying pan with a little oil and place over a medium-high heat. Add the sausages and onion and cook for 12–15 minutes, turning frequently, then remove to a chopping board.

Add the bacon and the mushrooms to the same pan and cook for 6–7 minutes, until crispy, then spoon on to the chopping board.

Slice the sausages and chop the bacon. Once the potatoes are cooked, add them to the frying pan.

Crack over the eggs into the four quarters of the pan, then add the bacon, mushrooms, onion and sausages on top. Cover with a lid and cook for 2–3 minutes (don't stir!), until the eggs are set.

Sprinkle the cheese and chives over the top, and serve.

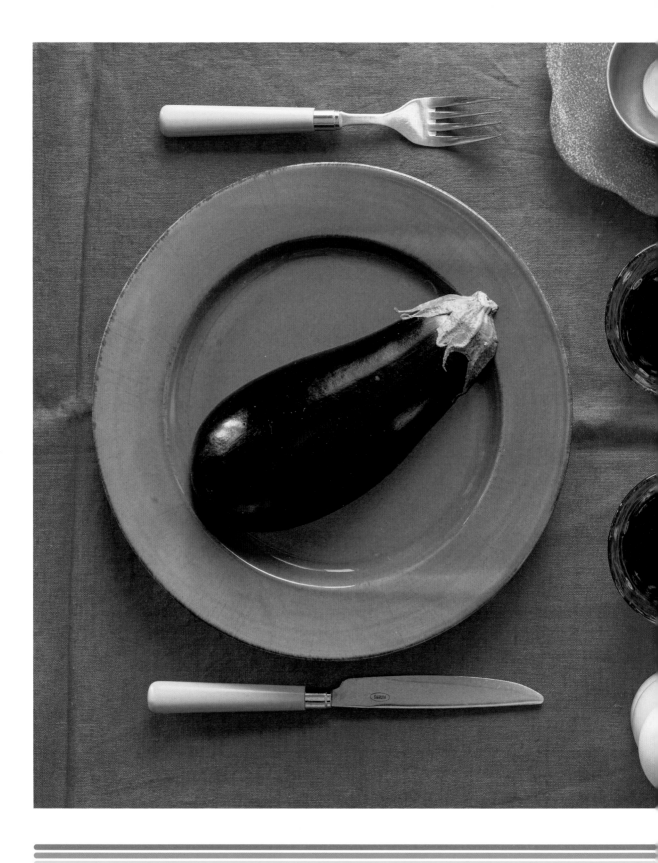

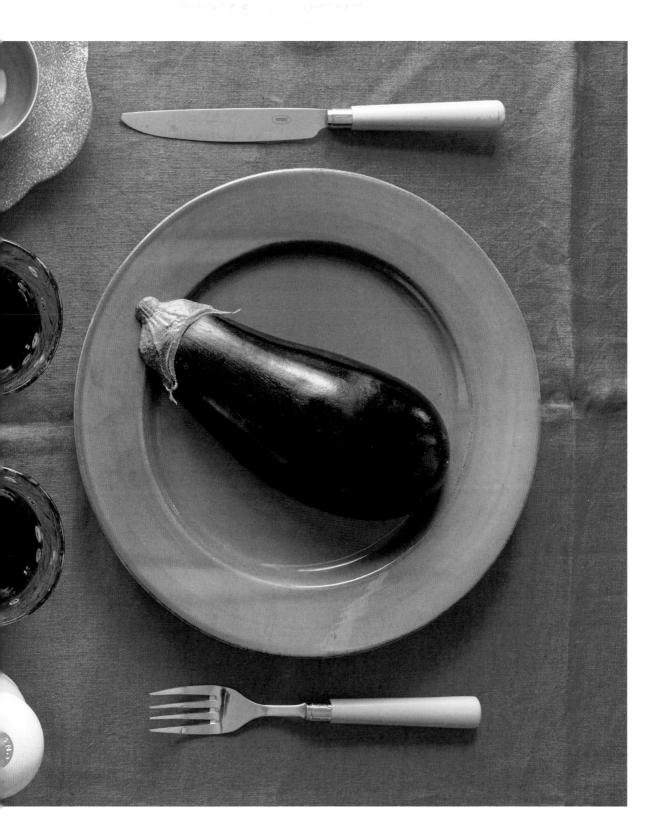

SALADS & SIDES

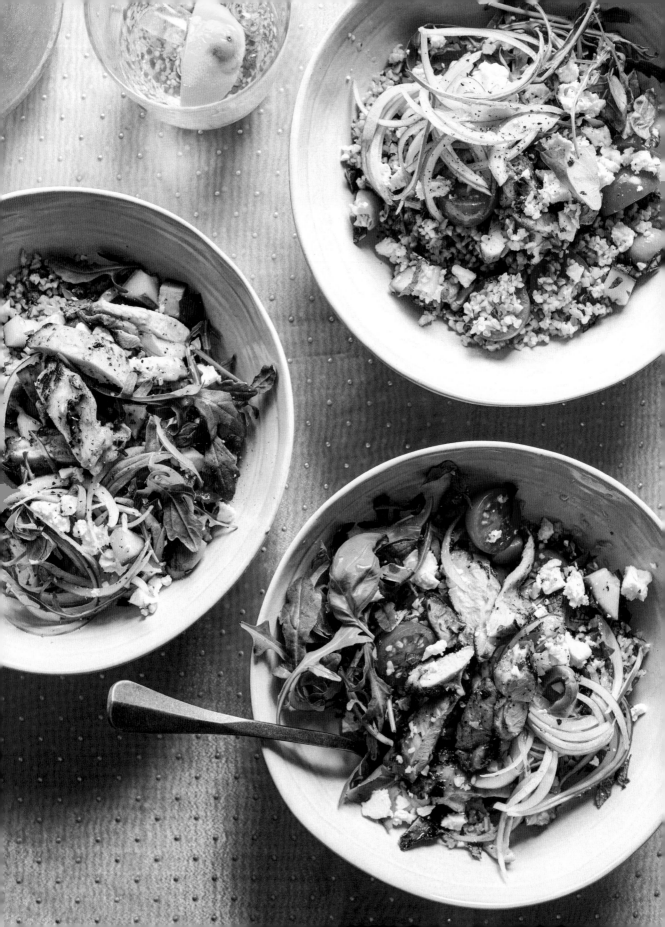

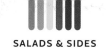
MEDITERRANEAN BUDDHA BOWL

The concept of a Buddha bowl has been around for some time now, and despite naked Paul and I looking exactly like those god-awful Buddha statues you sometimes see strewn about in posh garden centres, we have always swerved making any real attempt at them for the blog. If we are entirely honest, and I would like to think you and I are at the stage of our writer/reader relationship where we can be open about these things, the whole term seems like a bit of a nonsense. I mean, it's a salad in a bowl, let's not get ahead of ourselves.

But WHAT a salad – any combination of chicken, grain and other wonders is always going to be a winner. So please, although we are tipping our hat to the Buddha bowl trend and have subsequently photographed the food in a pleasingly fancy way, you should know that we could have just as easily called this one 'reet good chicken salad'.

Sidenote: who buys all those bloody awful statues anyway? Someone must, but if I peered out into our garden and saw some squat granite-faced goblin I'd just assume it was Paul.

SERVES: 4
PREP: 10 minutes
COOK: 10 minutes
CALORIES: 334

1 red onion
1 tablespoon red wine vinegar
100g (3½oz) bulgur wheat
2 teaspoons honey
zest and juice of ½ lemon
1 large bunch of fresh basil, chopped
1 large bunch of fresh mint, chopped
1 tablespoon olive oil
1 teaspoon salt
½ teaspoon black pepper
4 skinless, boneless chicken thighs
200g (7oz) cherry tomatoes, halved
½ a cucumber, deseeded and chopped
60g (2¼oz) rocket
60g (2¼oz) green olives, halved
100g (3½oz) reduced-fat feta, crumbled

Peel and thinly slice the onion, then place in a bowl with the red wine vinegar, stir, and set aside.

Bring 400ml (14fl oz) of water to the boil in a large pan and add the bulgur wheat. Stir, cover with a lid, reduce the heat to low and simmer for 15 minutes, then drain.

Meanwhile, mix together the honey, lemon zest and juice, half the basil and mint, the olive oil, salt and pepper, and rub over the chicken thighs.

Place a pan over a medium-high heat, add the chicken thighs with all their marinade, and cook for about 5 minutes each side, until browned. Remove to a board and roughly chop.

Serve the bulgur wheat in bowls and top with the tomatoes, cucumber, rocket, olives and chopped chicken.

Sprinkle over the pickled onion, feta and the remaining basil and mint.

NOTE

Couscous, farro, quinoa or even rice are great substitutes for the bulgur wheat.

BACON 'N' EGG SALAD

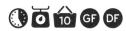

Bacon and egg salad: I'm not saying we are one of those tiresome internet pairs who wets their knickers over bacon or anything, but I can't deny we absolutely love the stuff. However, in the interests of making this fancy, we're swapping out bacon for Parma ham but please note that fat rashers of back bacon will do the job perfectly.

While I'm here picking apart Paul's recipe like the cruel monster that I am, Paul's a big fan of boiling an egg until you could drop it from the Eiffel Tower and comfortably hit the moon on the rebound. Though he has dialled back that particular tendency for this recipe, I'd suggest boiling the eggs for a minute less than we say: personal preference of course, but there's nothing more glorious than a wibbly-wobbly egg oozing yolk across your plate.

SERVES: 4
PREP: 5 minutes
COOK: 20 minutes
CALORIES: 245

4 eggs
2 large tins of new potatoes, drained
6 slices of Parma ham
2 shallots, sliced
2 tablespoons wholegrain mustard
3 tablespoons cider vinegar
300g (10½oz) mixed salad leaves
2 celery stalks, sliced

Bring a pan of water to the boil, add the eggs, and cook for 7 minutes. Remove the eggs from the pan and into a bowl of iced water for 5 minutes, then peel and set aside.

Meanwhile, dice the potatoes into 2cm (¾ inch) chunks and set aside.

Spray a frying pan with a little oil and place over a medium heat. Add the Parma ham to the pan and cook for 1 minute each side to crisp it up, then remove to a plate and roughly chop.

Spray the pan with a little more oil, then add the potatoes and cover with a lid. Cook for 5 minutes, shaking the pan regularly, then add the shallots. Cook for a further 5 minutes, then remove the pan from the heat.

Add the mustard and cider vinegar to the potatoes and stir well to mix.

Meanwhile, wash and pat dry the salad leaves. Toss with the celery and potatoes, then divide between four plates and top with the Parma ham.

Halve the eggs and add to each plate.

NOTE

Any salad leaves you want can be used for this – we like a mixture of spinach, rocket and lettuce, but it's entirely up to you!

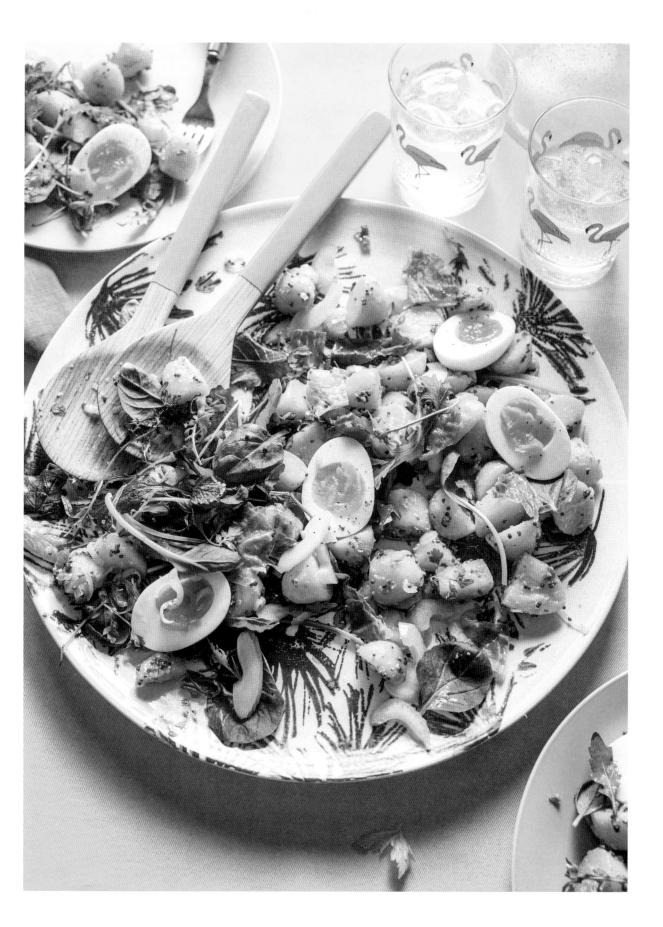

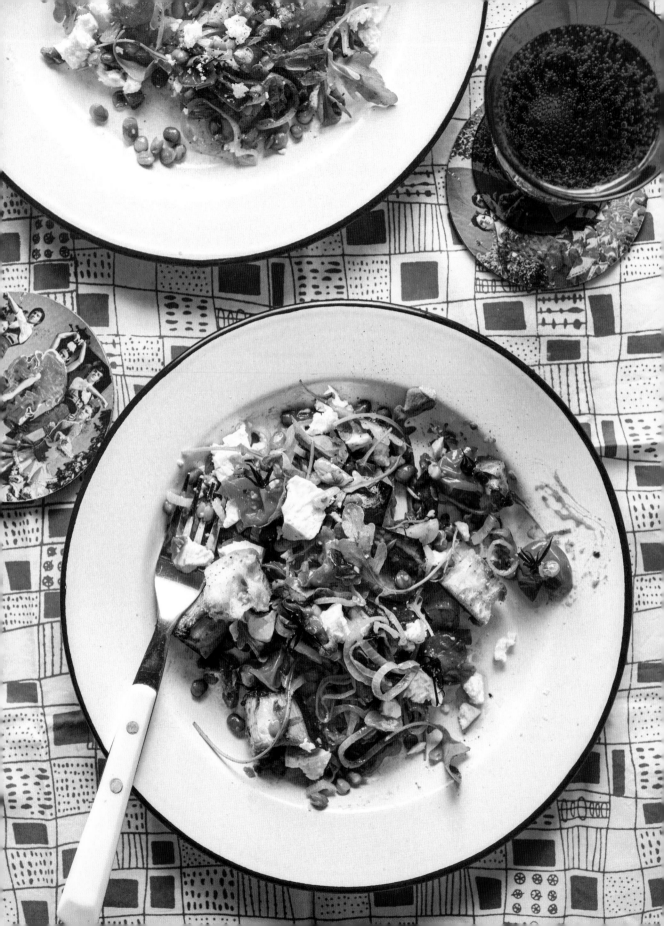

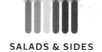
ROASTED TOMATO & LENTIL SALAD

Tomatoes: you know we love them, and here they are the star of the show. Well, I say we love them, Paul only tolerates them, but mind, I still have to tie his shoelaces for him so I think that tells you how much stock you should place next to his opinion.

Fair play to the man, though, he has come round to them over time, and that should be applauded. What is life without learning to love the things you used to hate? Admittedly that's an easy business when you're dealing with a dish as resplendent and nourishing as this one, but it does give me a moment of pause. After all, if Paul can grow to love tomatoes, does that mean there's a moment in my future where I'll look at pastel chinos and the idea of playing golf and consider either a good idea?

If that happens, please feel free to push me into the sea like Harold Bishop.

SERVES: 4
PREP: 10 minutes
COOK: 45 minutes
CALORIES: 310

2 aubergines
250g (9oz) cherry tomatoes
2 tablespoons balsamic vinegar
2 bread rolls
2 shallots, peeled and thinly
    sliced
2 cloves of garlic, crushed
    or grated
60g (2¼oz) sun-dried tomatoes,
    drained and chopped
1 × 390g (13½oz) tin of green
    lentils, drained
1 × 400g (14oz) tin of tomatoes,
    drained and rinsed (approx.
    230g/8¼oz)
80g (2¾oz) rocket
2 tablespoons red wine vinegar
150g (5½oz) reduced-fat feta
    cheese, crumbled

Preheat the oven to 220°C fan/475°F/gas mark 9.

Trim the aubergine, cut it in half lengthways, then chop into 2cm (¾ inch) pieces. Place the aubergine and tomatoes in a baking tray and spray with a little oil, then pour over the balsamic vinegar and toss.

Roast in the oven for 15–20 minutes, until softened and charred.

Meanwhile, cut the bread rolls into 2cm (¾ inch) chunks and place on another baking tray. Spray with a little oil, then bake in the oven for 8–10 minutes, to make the croutons.

Spray a large frying pan with a little oil and place over a medium-high heat. Add the shallots and fry for 2–3 minutes until soft, then add the garlic and sun-dried tomatoes.

Cook for another minute, and then add the lentils and stir. Reduce the heat to low and cook for 5–10 minutes, then remove from the heat.

Add the aubergine, tinned tomatoes and rocket to the lentils and stir to combine.

Sprinkle over the red wine vinegar and top with the croutons and feta.

CHICKEN CAESAR SALAD BOWL

This recipe came about in the great lockdown of 2020, when we were all stuck at home twiddling our thumbs and trying not to pitch heavy objects off our partner's heads. Just me? Either way, a friend of mine set up a Twitter competition known as Disaster Chef, where each week there would be a different theme and people would compete to win nothing more than some adulation and praise. Naturally, as a fiercely competitive person, I submitted this under the 'fancy' category and won. Joke was on me, though: I won a copy of my own book, signed by my hairy hand.

And I mean, I know where that hand has been.

Do give this a go, and don't be beholden to the salad I put inside. You can pretty much have anything you like in there, as long as it isn't too wet. And although the instructions may seem complex, they're really not. Think it through, pretend you're on *The Krypton Factor*, and this could be yours!

SERVES: 4
PREP: 10 minutes
COOK: 5 minutes
CALORIES: 409

1 ciabatta bun, halved
1 clove of garlic
200g (7oz) Parmesan cheese
200g (7oz) leftover chicken
   breast, chopped
1 large romaine lettuce,
   chopped fine
a handful of black olives
a drizzle of Caesar salad dressing

You will need two bowls of the same size that fit inside each other and some greaseproof paper.

Give the two halves of your ciabatta a little brush with oil, rub with the garlic, then grill until toasted and chop up for croutons.

Grate your Parmesan using the rough side of the grater (you don't want it too fine).

Pop a circle of greaseproof paper (bigger than the width of your bowls) on a plate and trace around the top of your bowl. Spread the Parmesan out so it covers the outline and a little over.

Microwave until the cheese has melted and crisped just a little.

Flip the cheesy paper so it covers an upside-down bowl, then put the other bowl on top – you're creating a sandwich with the cheese between the two bowls.

Allow to cool, then remove the bowls and the paper and set the cheese bowl aside to harden up.

Meanwhile, combine your chicken, lettuce and olives in a bowl.

Fill the cheese bowl with your salad, drizzle with the Caesar salad dressing. Split in half and break off bits as you go to enjoy. You could even be disgustingly romantic and share your salad bowl and plate …

NOTES

If you wanted to be a total smart-a*se about things, you could whittle yourself a knife and fork from breadsticks, but let's not be that person, eh?

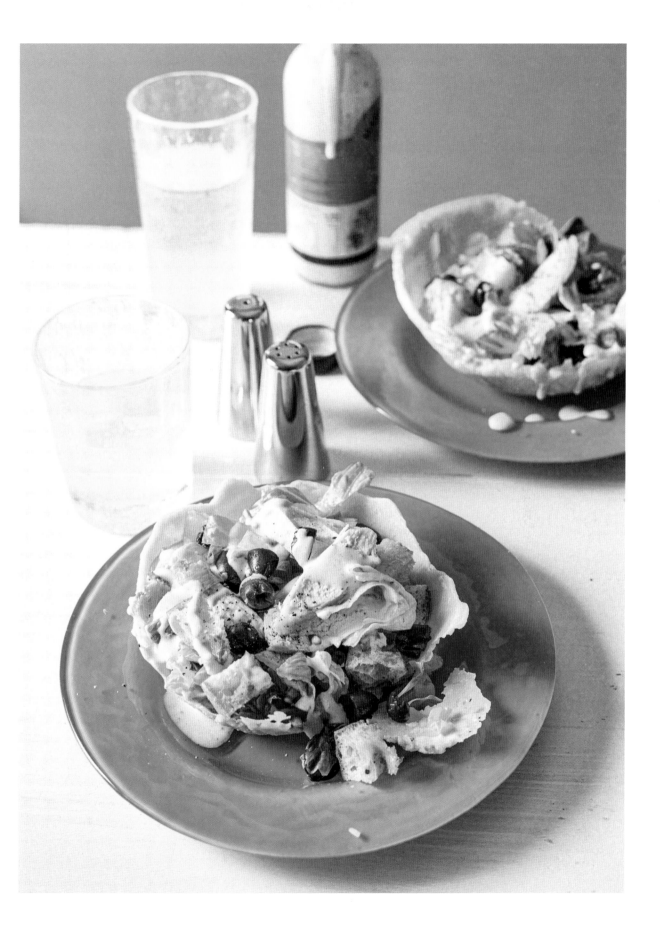

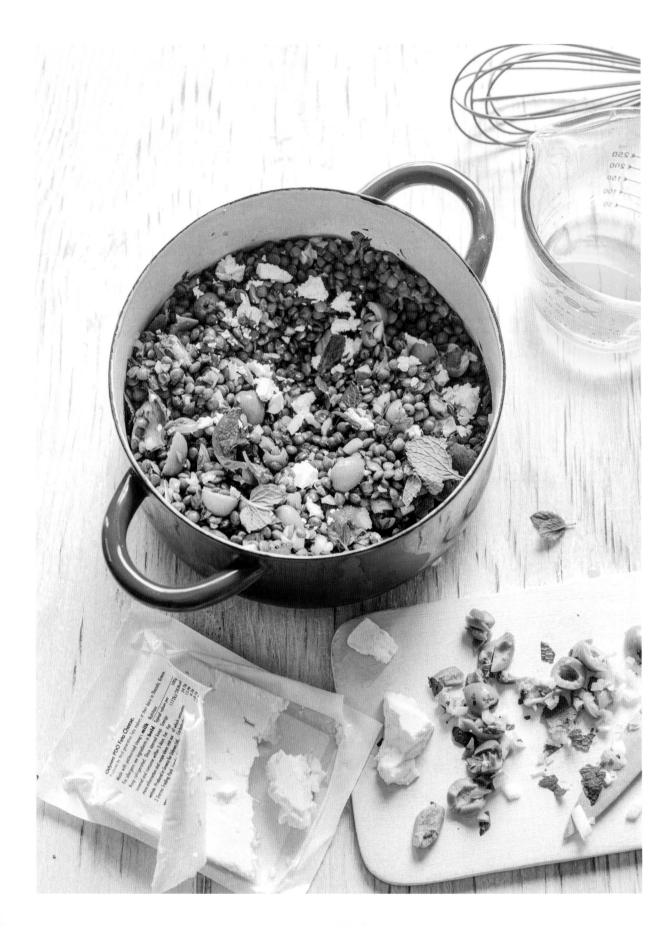

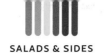
MEDITERRANEAN LENTIL SALAD

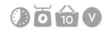

Lentils remain one of those ingredients that I never have enough trust in: I always imagine they'll tumble on to the dinner plate and be devoid of all flavour and happiness, and readers, I'm forever wrong. Cooked smartly and with care, mixing with all sorts of deliciousness, they can be a joy – and never more so than in this lentil salad, which provides a very full, hearty meal indeed. Plus: it's a salad, so you know what that means, don't you? A full-size airport-bought duty-free Toblerone for dessert because you've saved those calories. Together, we're winning at dieting!

I should trust more, I know. It would certainly make my life easier – I don't even trust the reversing sensors on my car, and I paid extra for them when I bought it. To be fair to me, though, I've seen how Skynet starts and we all know how terribly mean AI can be, so I'm sure malevolently shunting my little Golf into our garden wall is high on the robotic agenda. No, I'll stick to getting a crick in my neck and shouting as I reverse, thank you very much.

SERVES: 4
PREP: 1 hour 10 minutes
COOK: 45 minutes
CALORIES: 315

220g (8oz) dried green lentils, rinsed
1 teaspoon salt
400ml (14fl oz) vegetable stock
5 cloves of garlic, crushed
1 bay leaf
3 tablespoons olive oil
3 tablespoons white wine vinegar
90g (3¼oz) pitted olives, roughly chopped
15g (½oz) fresh mint leaves, chopped
1 large shallot, finely diced
30g (1oz) feta cheese

Put the lentils into a bowl with the salt. Cover with 1 litre (1¾ pints) of warm water and leave to soak for 1 hour, then drain.

Preheat the oven to 170°C fan/375°F/gas mark 5.

Put the lentils, stock, garlic and bay leaf into a lidded ovenproof saucepan or casserole dish and cook in the oven for 45 minutes. Drain the lentils again, discarding the liquid, and remove the bay leaf.

Whisk together the olive oil and white wine vinegar to make a dressing.

Put the lentils back into the pan, add the olives, mint and shallots and pour over the dressing.

Crumble over the feta and serve.

NOTE

In a hurry? Tinned lentils, or lentils from a pouch, will do – simply heat and mix together with the olives, mint, shallots and feta – but soaking your own lentils does help get the best texture and the best taste, and is really cheap.

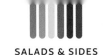
VEG 5 WAYS

This book is full of wonderful dinner ideas, but sometimes you need a bit on the side. Just don't tell Paul. So to satisfy those little urges, we're including here five wonderful little side dishes that will complement all the meals so far. We say this with a caution though – and please forgive us our scurrility – if you think your post-sprout toots are enough to be ashamed about, wait until you add spice into the mix.

SPANISH-STYLE STEWED TOMATOES & PEPPERS

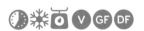

See dish 1, page 162

SERVES: 4 as a side
PREP: 5 minutes
COOK: 50 minutes
CALORIES: 76

1 tablespoon olive oil
1 red onion, sliced
2 cloves of garlic, sliced
2 red peppers, sliced into 2cm (¾ inch) strips
3 plum tomatoes, roughly chopped
1 teaspoon sweet smoked paprika
a splash of sherry or red wine vinegar
2 teaspoons capers, drained
2 tablespoons chopped fresh flat-leaf parsley
salt and black pepper

Heat the oil in a medium pan. Add the red onion and cook for 7–8 minutes. Add the garlic and cook for a further 2 minutes, then add the peppers, tomatoes and paprika, and season with salt and pepper. Stir thoroughly, then pop a lid on. Leave on a medium-low heat for 35–40 minutes, stirring regularly until the peppers are soft. Add a splash of vinegar to taste, and season well.

Serve topped with the capers and parsley.

SPICY SZECHUAN-ESQUE CABBAGE

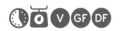

See dish 2, page 162

SERVES: 4 as a side
PREP: 3 minutes
COOK: 10 minutes
CALORIES: 149

1 sweetheart cabbage
1–2 tablespoons vegetable oil
1 teaspoon Sichuan peppercorns, bashed
2–3 dried red chillies
3 cloves of garlic, sliced
1 tablespoon soy sauce or tamari
1 tablespoon sugar

Cut the cabbage into 8 wedges lengthways, removing the core, then into large chunks widthways.

Heat the oil in a wok or a large non-stick frying pan. Add the peppercorns and chillies and toast in the oil for 1 minute. Add the garlic for a further minute.

Add the cabbage and stir-fry for 6–7 minutes, or until tender but still with some bite. Be sure to stir it frequently so the garlic doesn't burn.

Mix together the soy sauce and sugar. Pour into the cabbage, stir, and remove from the heat. Serve hot.

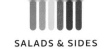
GREEN SALAD

 V GF

See dish 3, page 163

SERVES: 4 as a side
PREP: 5 minutes
CALORIES: 146

2 little gem lettuces
50g (1¾oz) rocket
1 baby cucumber (or ½ a large
    one), halved and sliced
4 celery stalks, sliced thinly
40g (1½oz) Parmesan or
    vegetarian Italian-style hard
    cheese

For the dressing
3 tablespoons extra virgin olive oil
juice of ½ lemon
1 teaspoon Dijon mustard
a small handful of fresh dill,
    chopped
salt and black pepper

Separate the leaves of the little gems and put them into a large salad bowl with the rocket, cucumber and celery.

In a jar, mix together the dressing ingredients along with half the dill. Toss through the salad, then top with the remaining dill. Use a peeler to shave the Parmesan over the top, then season and serve.

CRISPY HAM & CREAMY PEAS

See dish 4, page 163

SERVES: 4 as a side
PREP: 3 minutes
COOK: 7 minutes
CALORIES: 108

3 slices of Parma ham
300g (10½oz) frozen peas
75g (2½oz) low-fat cream cheese
zest of 1 lemon and juice, to taste
salt and black pepper

Heat a non-stick pan over a medium heat and add the ham. Cook for 2–3 minutes, or until crisp, turning halfway through. Set aside to cool, then chop roughly.

Blanch the peas in boiling water until defrosted, then drain and return to the pan. Stir through the cream cheese over a low heat until it melts through. Add the lemon zest and a squeeze of lemon, and season to taste. Serve hot, topped with the Parma ham.

ROAST CHILLI SPROUTS

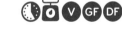 V GF DF

See dish 5, page 163

SERVES: 4 as a side
PREP: 5 minutes
COOK: 25 minutes
CALORIES: 92

500g (1lb 2oz) Brussels sprouts
1 tablespoon olive oil
¼ teaspoon chilli flakes
salt

Preheat the oven to 200°C fan/425°F/gas mark 7.

Trim the base of the sprouts and remove any tough outer leaves. Halve the sprouts and put them on a baking tray. Add the oil and toss lightly. Sprinkle with the chilli flakes and salt, then bake for 20–25 minutes or until golden, tossing the sprouts every 10 minutes.

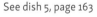

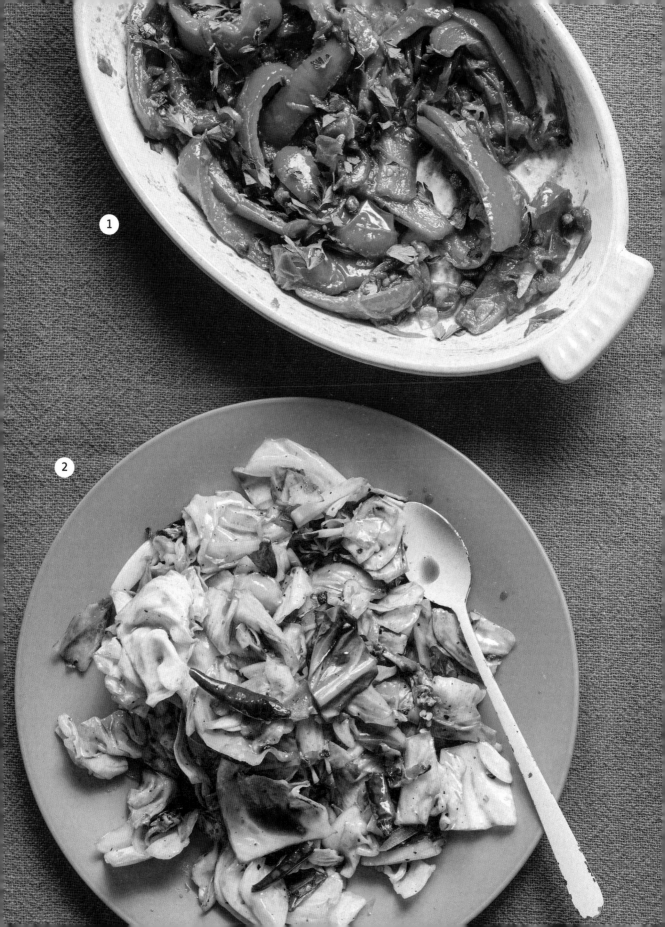

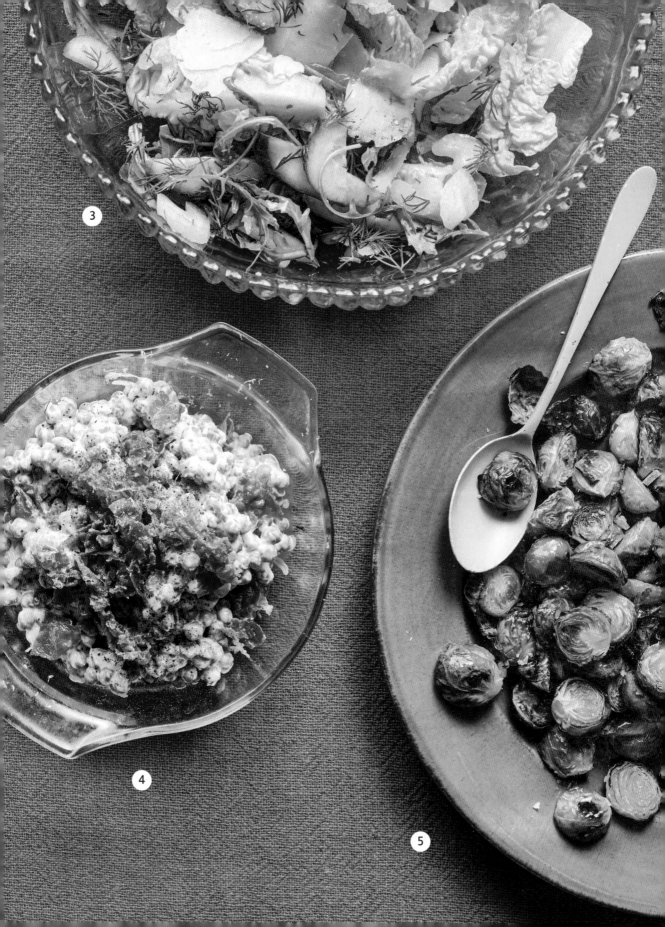

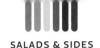
KAPUSTA PIEROGI

We adore pierogi. Adore them. We may not be able to confidently spell the word without double-checking, and I can't in all good conscience say we are absolutely certain even now, but they're just incredible. We were lucky enough to sneak a weekend away in Krakow before the various COVID lockdowns of 2020 hit, and it skyrocketed up our favourite places in the world: a beautiful city with wonderful food and men that makes your thighs quake.

As part of our weekend we took lunch in a little café hidden down the back streets recommended to us on our Facebook page and had I dropped down dead right there, I'd have died a happy man. They kept bringing little plates of these pierogi, stuffed with all sorts of different flavours, and each one was delicious. Not delicious was the warm mulled beer that accompanied them. But even that couldn't derail what was the best hour of that holiday.

And listen, we spend a good proportion of any holiday excitedly pushing meaty parcels over our lips so this is high praise. Let this be our gift to you – each pierogi has 22 calories.

MAKES: about 40 pierogi
PREP: 30 minutes
COOK: 55 minutes
CALORIES: 22 per pierogi

1 onion, finely diced
200g (7oz) sauerkraut, drained
3 large porcini mushrooms, finely diced
1 tablespoon panko breadcrumbs
165g (5¾oz) plain flour
1 teaspoon salt
1 tablespoon butter
90ml (3fl oz) warm water
black pepper

Spray a saucepan with a little oil and place over a medium-low heat. Add the onion and cook for 5–6 minutes, until softened.

Add the sauerkraut, mushrooms and a pinch of salt and pepper and stir. Cover the pan with a lid and simmer for 40 minutes, stirring occasionally. Add a splash of water if it starts to stick.

Take the pan off the heat. Remove one-third of the mixture to a blender or food processor, blitz until smooth, then return to the pan. Add the panko breadcrumbs and stir well, then set aside.

Put the flour into a bowl with the salt and make a well in the middle. Add the butter and gently cut it into the dough, gradually adding the warm water as you go.

Mix and knead the dough for 5 minutes, until smooth and soft. Cover the bowl with a tea towel and leave for 20 minutes.

Divide the dough in half. Slap one half out on to a floured surface and roll out to about 2–3mm thick. Use a 7cm biscuit cutter to cut out as many circles of dough as you can, using any excess to roll out a new sheet. Cover them with a tea towel, then repeat with the other half of the dough (you should get about 40 circles in total).

Spoon 1 teaspoon of the sauerkraut mix into the centre of each dough circle, then fold into a half-moon shape and crimp the edges to seal.

Bring a large pan of water to the boil. Add up to 15 pierogi at a time to the pan, boil for 4–5 minutes until they float to the top, then remove to a plate and serve.

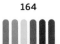

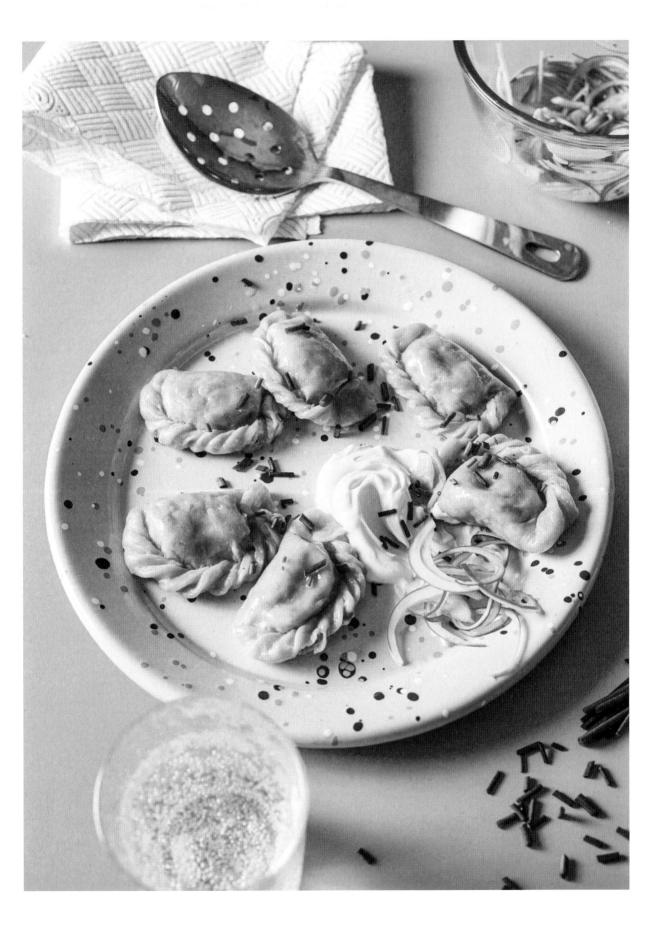

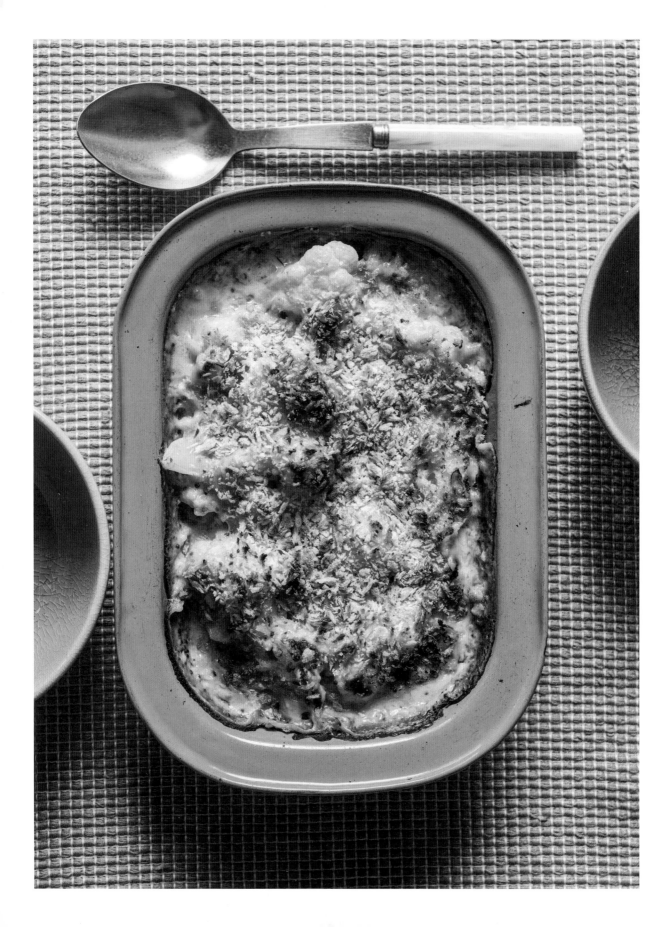

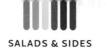

CAULIFLOWER CHEESE

While we have tried to include some more unusual dishes this time around, sometimes it's the simple dinners that win your heart. Cauliflower cheese is a personal favourite of mine, although Paul doesn't quite trust cauliflower enough to fully submit to this: he sees it as vampire broccoli, and although he might be right, he's missing out terribly here. Of course, as it is us, the recipe is slightly more advanced than your bog-standard cauliflower cheese, but there's nothing in there that should cause too much consternation.

A little tip: the sharper the cheese, the better the dish. None of this mild Cheddar muck, which has absolutely no place in cooking, ever. Marks & Spencer do my absolute favourite cheese – Cornish Cruncher – and I encourage you to seek it out if you haven't tried it. We aren't getting paid to promote, but should the chiefs at M&S fancy sending us a crate to work through, please note we will accept such a trouble willingly.

SERVES: 4
PREP: 10 minutes
COOK: 45 minutes
CALORIES: 328

1 large cauliflower, cut into florets
1 onion, finely sliced
3 bacon medallions, finely diced
2 cloves of garlic, crushed
¼ teaspoon paprika
40g (1½oz) plain flour
500ml (18fl oz) skimmed milk
1½ tablespoons wholegrain
   mustard
125g (4½oz) reduced-fat mature
   Cheddar cheese, grated
25g (1oz) panko breadcrumbs

Preheat the oven to 200°C fan/425°F/gas mark 7.

Bring a large saucepan of water to the boil. Add the cauliflower and cook for 5 minutes, then drain and tip into an ovenproof dish.

Meanwhile, spray a large frying pan with a little oil and place over a medium heat. Add the onion and cook for 10 minutes, until softened. Add the bacon and cook for another 5 minutes, until crispy.

Add the garlic, paprika and flour and cook for another minute. Slowly pour the milk into the pan, stirring continuously, until it thickens. Add the mustard and Cheddar and give another good stir.

Pour the cheese sauce over the cauliflower and give a gentle stir.

Sprinkle over the panko breadcrumbs and bake in the oven for 25 minutes until golden.

NOTES

Leave out the bacon if you want to make this more traditional, or veggie – it's just as good!

Swap out half the cauliflower for broccoli if you fancy mixing it up a bit.

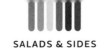
POTATOES 5 WAYS

We know we did a batch of potato ideas in book one and so another pentad of potato recipes may seem an indulgence but hear us out: everyone loves potatoes. And those that don't, well, there's no accounting for taste (but we're sure you're lovely). They're cheap, they're easy to cook with and they carry so much flavour when cooked right. Plus it's a well known fact that potatoes make for great detectives. Why? Because they always keep their eyes peeled.

I'll see myself out.

WHOLE PAN SQUEAK

See dish 1, page 170

SERVES: 4
PREP: 5 minutes
COOK: 20 minutes
CALORIES: 334

1 tablespoon olive oil
3 rashers of streaky bacon, chopped
1 red onion, finely chopped
170g (6oz) cooked cabbage or other Sunday greens
100g (3½oz) mature Cheddar cheese
500g (1lb 2oz) leftover mashed potatoes
salt and black pepper

Heat a medium frying pan over a medium heat. Add the oil, then the bacon and onion. Fry for 5 minutes, then add the cooked cabbage (or other greens). Cook for a further 3–4 minutes to get a little colour, stirring everything together.

Grate the Cheddar into the mash and mix together. Add the potato mixture to the pan, stir everything together, then press the mixture into the pan firmly. Cook over a medium heat for about 6–8 minutes, until the base is firm and crisp. Flip it over on to a plate, then cut into chunky wedges and serve.

BOMBAY-ISH POTATOES

See dish 2, page 170

SERVES: 4
PREP: 10 minutes
COOK: 30 minutes
CALORIES: 223

900g (2lb) Maris Piper potatoes
olive oil
2 banana shallots
1 tablespoon cumin seeds
2 teaspoons chilli powder
1 teaspoon ground turmeric
1 teaspoon mustard seeds
1 teaspoon black onion seeds
1 × 400g (14oz) tin of chopped tomatoes
a handful of fresh coriander, chopped
salt and black pepper

Peel the potatoes and cut into 4cm (1½ inch) chunks. Boil them in salted water until tender and let them steam dry in a colander.

Heat a little oil in a medium pan. Add the shallots and cook for 5 minutes, then add the spices and cook for another 2 minutes. Add a little more oil to the pan, then add the potatoes, stirring so they are nicely coated, and cook for a further 2–3 minutes. Don't worry if the potatoes break up a little bit. Season with salt and pepper.

Add the tinned tomatoes and cook for a further 15–20 minutes, or until thick. Stir through the coriander before serving.

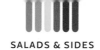
SALT & PEPPER POTATO DISCS

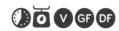

See dish 3, page 171

SERVES: 4
PREP: 5 minutes
COOK: 30 minutes
CALORIES: 215

750g (1lb 10oz) Maris Piper potatoes
2 tablespoons vegetable oil
salt and lots of black pepper

Preheat the oven to 200°C fan/425°F/gas mark 7.

Peel the potatoes and thinly slice them about 2mm (¹⁄₁₆ inch) thick. Line two large baking trays with baking paper, drizzle with a thin layer of oil and spread out the potatoes – it's OK for them to overlap a little. Sprinkle with plenty of salt.

Bake for 20–30 minutes or until crispy, checking on the potatoes every 10 minutes or so to turn them or remove the ones that are ready.

Remove from the oven, add lots of black pepper, and serve.

GLAZED SWEET POTATOES

See dish 4, page 171

SERVES: 4
PREP: 5 minutes
COOK: 40 minutes
CALORIES: 155

2 sweet potatoes
olive oil
1 tablespoon maple syrup
1 tablespoon chopped rosemary
salt

Preheat the oven to 180°C fan/400°F/gas mark 6.

Peel the potatoes and slice into 1cm (½ inch) discs. Brush with olive oil, sprinkle with salt and bake for 25–30 minutes, until tender and a little golden, turning over once during the cooking time.

Remove the tray from the oven and brush the potatoes with the maple syrup. Sprinkle over the rosemary and bake for a further 5–10 minutes, or until sticky and golden.

MEXICAN POTATO SALAD

See dish 5, page 171

SERVES: 4
PREP: 10 minutes
COOK: 10 minutes
CALORIES: 366

700g (1lb 9oz) new potatoes
2 corn on the cob
3 tablespoons low-fat mayo
juice of ½ lime
2 tablespoons chopped pickled jalapeños
2 avocados, cut into cubes
a handful of fresh coriander, chopped
salt and black pepper

Preheat the grill to high.

Cut the potatoes into 3cm (1¼ inch) chunks and boil in salted water until tender, about 10 minutes. In the meantime, strip the corn kernels off their husks, spread them out on a tray and grill for 10 minutes, turning over halfway through the cooking time.

Drain the potatoes and set aside. When cool, add the corn to the potatoes. Mix the mayonnaise with the lime juice, season well with salt and pepper, and stir in the chopped jalapeños. Toss to coat the potatoes and corn, then finally stir through the avocado and coriander and serve.

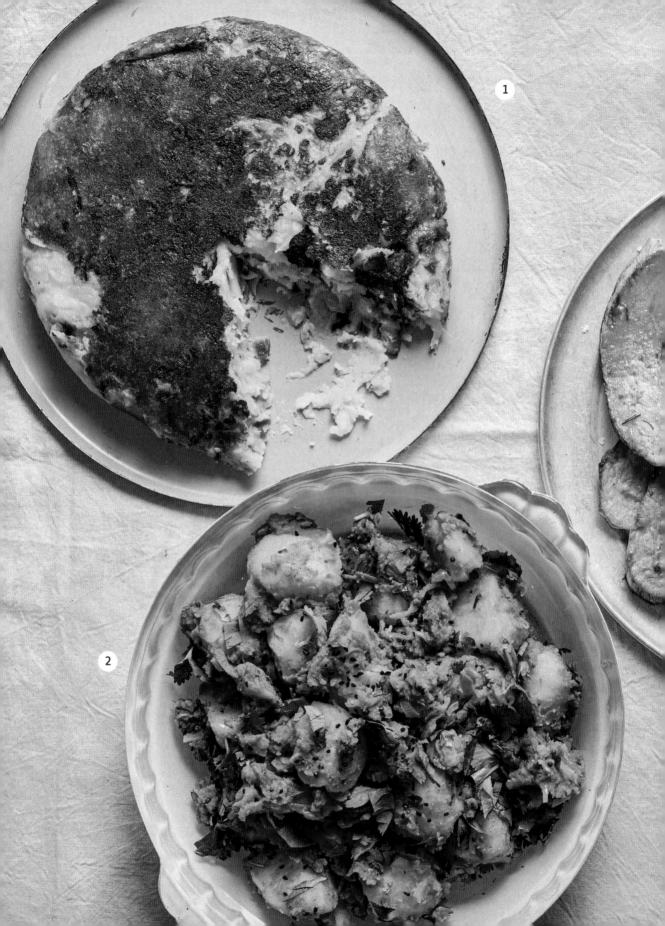

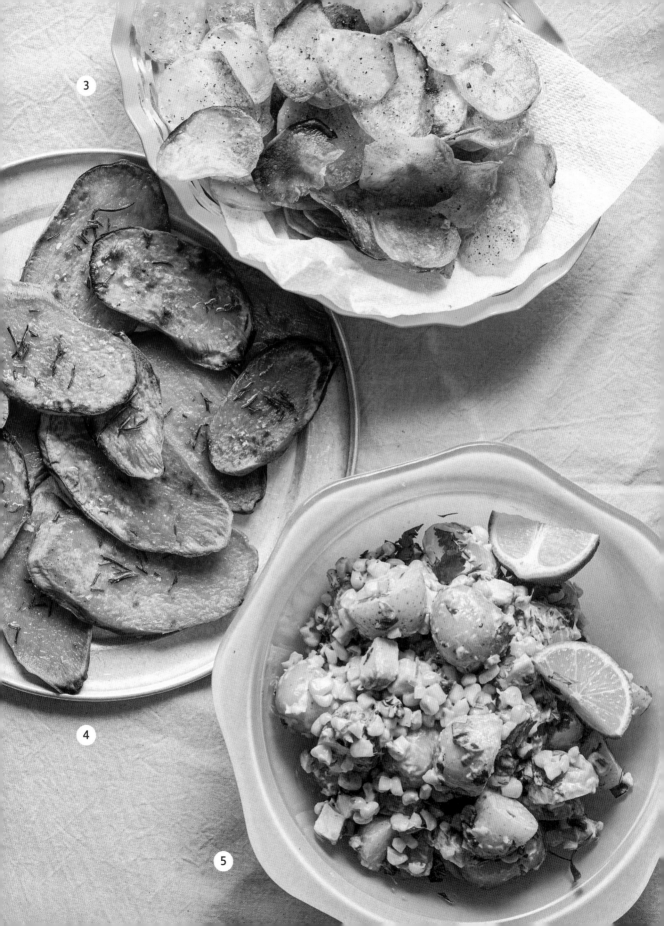

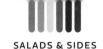

KOREAN CHICKEN BITES

Another holiday recipe this one: can you tell how easily influenced we are by our bellies? Neither of us can remember exactly where we were country-wise when we had these, but both remember being sat at a very classy bar on those high stools that show your a*se-crack to everyone sitting behind you when we were served these as bar-snacks. I mean, they're delicious, but anything covered in drippy sticky sauce is never suitable as finger-food.

Paul demonstrated this in his usual way by taking one bite and immediately cascading the rest all down one of my favourite shirts. It's a trait of his I cannot fathom: he wears his own shirts for at least a decade without incident but the very second he slips something of mine on, stains and slicks appear as though he's keeping a gravy reservoir behind each ear. It's lucky I adore him (and know his PIN number so I can order a new shirt on his bank card).

Please do give these a go, though: they're unbelievably wonderful.

SERVES: 4
PREP: 10 minutes
COOK: 25 minutes
CALORIES: 426

2 tablespoons plain flour
½ teaspoon salt
¼ teaspoon black pepper
¼ teaspoon garlic granules
2 eggs
120g (4½oz) panko breadcrumbs
4 skinless, boneless chicken
    breasts, cut into chunks
3 spring onions, sliced thinly
1 teaspoon sesame seeds
½ teaspoon chilli flakes

For the sauce
1 tablespoon sriracha
1 tablespoon tomato purée
1 tablespoon honey
2 tablespoons brown sugar
4 tablespoons soy sauce
3 cloves of garlic, crushed
2 teaspoons grated root ginger
1 tablespoon sesame oil

Preheat the oven to 200°C fan/425°F/gas mark 7 and line a baking tray with greaseproof paper.

Mix together the flour, salt, pepper and garlic granules and pour into a shallow dish. Beat the eggs and place in another shallow dish, and pour the panko breadcrumbs into another.

In small batches, dredge the chicken in the flour, then dip in the egg and finally coat in the panko breadcrumbs (press it in if it's having trouble sticking). Place on the baking tray and repeat until all the chicken is breaded.

Bake in the oven for 15–20 minutes, until nicely golden.

While the chicken is cooking, put all the sauce ingredients into a saucepan and place over a medium-high heat. Bring to the boil, then simmer for 5 minutes until thickened.

When the chicken is cooked, remove from the oven and pour over the sauce.

Finally, sprinkle over the spring onions, sesame seeds and chilli flakes.

NOTE

We use sriracha and tomato purée as a cheaper alternative to the proper gochujang paste, but by all means if you can find it, use that instead (same quantity). Our version, though, is just as good and not as much of a ball-ache to find.

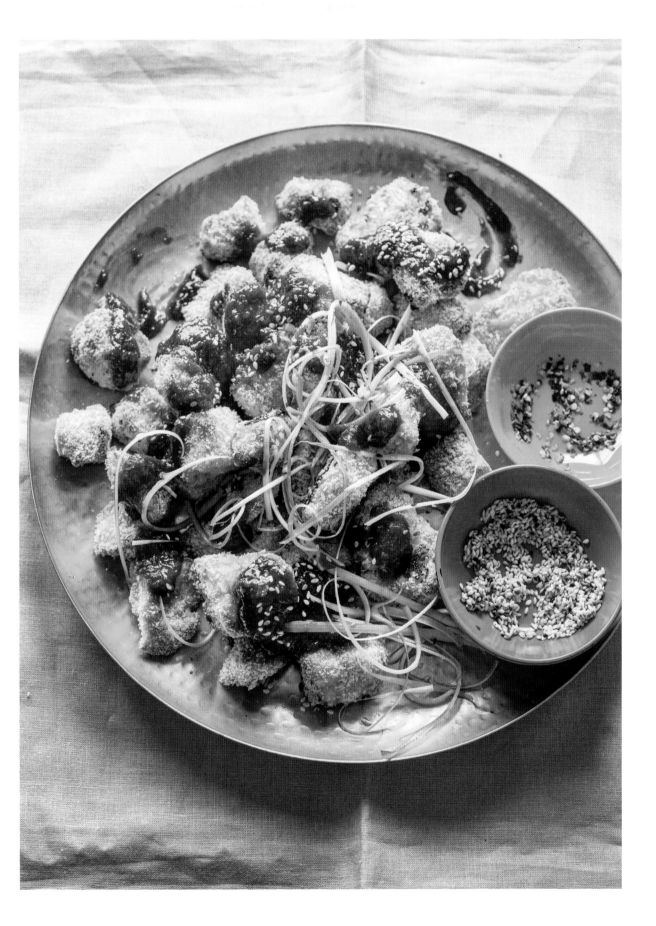

SPICY SQUASH & CAULIFLOWER

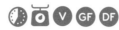

One of the casualties of our house fire was our dear, dear shed, which disappeared in a fiery blaze. We mourn that shed and the many treasures within, and although we've taken to enjoying the space outside where it used to be, I do so long for somewhere I can store everything that 'I need to find a home for' again. Paul's promised me a trip to Homebase in my future, but we all know that day isn't going to come. Hey, though, fun fact: a blazing fire will destroy all manner of things, but a sack of popcorn kernels? Entirely indestructible apparently!

A further victim of the blaze was the little vegetable patch I was quietly cultivating in the garden behind it, which I only raise because cauliflowers and potatoes were the only thing I ever managed to grow there. I did once cut the top off a pineapple and bury it in the garden in order to persuade Paul that pineapples will cheerfully grow in the inclement weather of Northumberland, and to his eternal discredit he believed me. I'd judge him, but I was thirty-five when I realised that pineapples don't grow high up on the trees like coconuts.

Anyhoo. If you have some cauliflower and want something different, do try this squash and cauliflower extravaganza. £100 that that's the first time 'extravaganza' and 'cauliflower' have ever been laid together in a sentence.

SERVES: 4
PREP: 15 minutes
COOK: 20 minutes
CALORIES: 290

1 cauliflower, cut into florets
1 butternut squash, peeled and cut into cubes
1 apple, diced
1 onion, peeled and cut into wedges
1 × 400g (14oz) tin of chickpeas, drained and rinsed
2½cm (1 inch) piece of ginger, grated
1 teaspoon ground turmeric
1 teaspoon garam masala
1 teaspoon paprika
1 teaspoon ground fennel seeds
1 teaspoon salt
2 tablespoons pumpkin seeds
3 tablespoons olive oil
3 tablespoons lime juice

Preheat the oven to 200°C fan/425°F/gas mark 7.

Put all the ingredients together into a bowl and toss together until well combined.

Spread them all out on a baking sheet and bake in the oven for 20 minutes until cooked through.

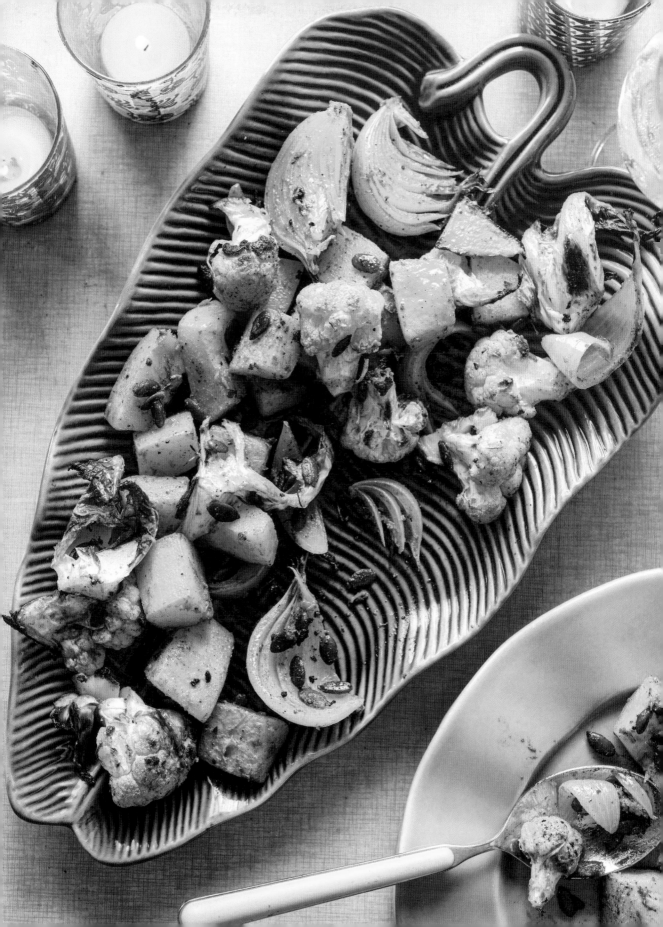

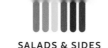

RICE 5 WAYS

Continuing our theme of five extra recipes to bring you glee and wonder, please find below five delicious things to do with rice. A lot of you seem to have the heebie-jeebies about cooking rice and you mustn't worry for a moment more, it's really terrifically easy. Of course, no matter how exact your measurements and how precise your cooking, you will end up with enough leftover rice to build a starchy igloo with. Listen, we don't make the rules.

GARLIC BUTTERED RICE

See dish 1, page 178

SERVES: 4
PREP: 5 minutes
COOK: 15 minutes
CALORIES: 287

1 tablespoon butter
1 tablespoon vegetable oil
4 plump cloves of garlic, thinly sliced
250g (9oz) long-grain rice
1 tablespoon dried parsley
salt and black pepper

Heat the butter and oil in a pan over a medium heat. Once the butter is melted and foaming, add the garlic and cook until golden and crispy (watch out as it can suddenly burn quickly). Scoop the garlic out, drain on a piece of kitchen paper, and season with salt.

Rinse the rice, add to the butter and oil and stir through, then add 500ml (18fl oz) of boiling water. Simmer for 9–12 minutes over a low heat with the lid on, until tender. Remove from the heat, then put a clean tea towel under the lid and leave to steam for a few minutes. Fluff up with a fork, then stir through the parsley and season. Serve with the garlic chips scattered over the top.

SPICY PILAF WITH YOGHURT & FLAKED ALMONDS

See dish 2, page 178

SERVES: 4
PREP: 5 minutes
COOK: 25 minutes
CALORIES: 348

1 tablespoon vegetable oil
2 shallots, sliced
2 tablespoons Madras curry paste
250g (9oz) long-grain rice
500ml (18fl oz) hot vegetable stock
4 tablespoons yoghurt
a handful of flaked almonds, toasted
a small handful of fresh coriander, chopped

Heat the oil. Add the shallots and cook for 5–10 minutes. Add the curry paste and cook for 2 minutes.

Rinse the rice and add to the pan, stirring to coat, then pour over the hot stock. Bring to a simmer with the lid on, then lower the heat and cook for 9–12 minutes (or until tender and the liquid is absorbed). Remove from the heat, pop a clean tea towel under the lid and leave to steam. Fluff up with a fork, and serve dolloped with the yoghurt and sprinkled with the almonds and coriander.

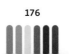

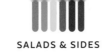
EGG FRIED RICE

See dish 3, page 179

SERVES: 4
REST: Overnight or
a few hours in fridge
PREP: 5 minutes
COOK: 15 minutes
CALORIES: 261

125g (4½oz) basmati rice
2 tablespoons sesame oil
3 cloves of garlic, sliced
4 eggs
150g (5½oz) frozen peas, thawed
4 spring onions, thinly sliced
soy sauce or salt

Start by cooking the rice if you don't have any leftovers, ideally the day before. Measure out the rice, then rinse until the water runs clear. Cook according to packet instructions. Fluff up the rice with a fork and spread out in a dish, then leave in the fridge to cool.

Heat a large non-stick pan. Add the sesame oil, then add the garlic. Sizzle for 1 minute, then push the garlic to one side of the pan and tilt the pan. Break the eggs into the oily part of the pan and use a wooden spoon to scramble them in the oil. Once cooked through, lay the pan flat again on the heat and add the rice. Stir regularly for 3–4 minutes, then add the peas. Stir again, and season well with soy sauce or salt. Finally stir through the spring onions and serve.

NUTTY WILD RICE SALAD

See dish 4, page 179

SERVES: 4
PREP: 5 minutes
COOK: 40 minutes
CALORIES: 407

200g (7oz) wild rice (black or red
    or a mix will work well)
90g (3¼oz) hazelnuts
50g (1¾oz) dried cranberries
a handful of fresh parsley, finely
    chopped
1 tablespoon extra virgin olive oil
juice of ½ lemon
salt and black pepper

Cook the rice according to the packet instructions, usually around 35–40 minutes. It should be still a bit al dente. In the meantime, toast the hazelnuts and roughly chop.

Soak the dried cranberries in a little boiling water. Drain after 5 minutes.

Once the rice is cooked, drain well. Leave to cool a little, then add the hazelnuts and cranberries, and stir through the parsley. Drizzle the oil and lemon juice over the top, season and serve.

RED RICE

See dish 5, page 179

SERVES: 4
PREP: 5 minutes
COOK: 35 minutes
CALORIES: 238

1 tablespoon olive oil
1 onion, diced
1 teaspoon sweet smoked paprika
1 tablespoon tomato purée
175g (6oz) paella or arborio rice
½ a glass of white wine
500ml (18fl oz) vegetable stock
200ml (7fl oz) passata
salt and black pepper

Heat the oil in a large pan. Add the onion and fry for 8–10 minutes, until soft and translucent.

Add the paprika and the tomato purée. Cook for 2 minutes, stirring often, then add the rice. Toast the rice for 2 minutes, then add the wine. Simmer until it evaporates, then add the vegetable stock and passata. Bring to a simmer over a low heat for 15–20 minutes, stirring every 5 or so minutes, until the rice is tender. Season to taste, and serve.

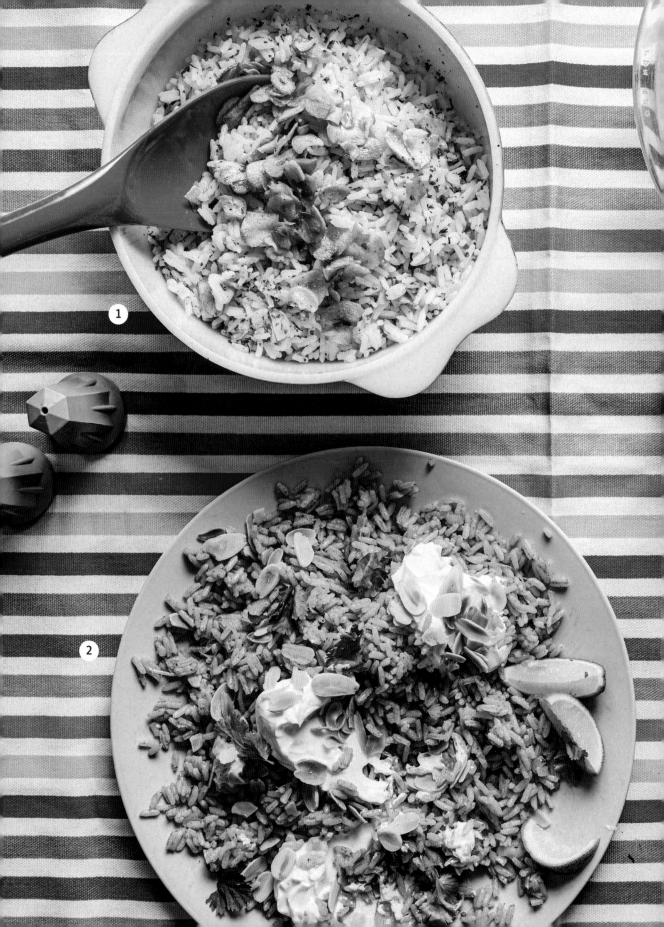

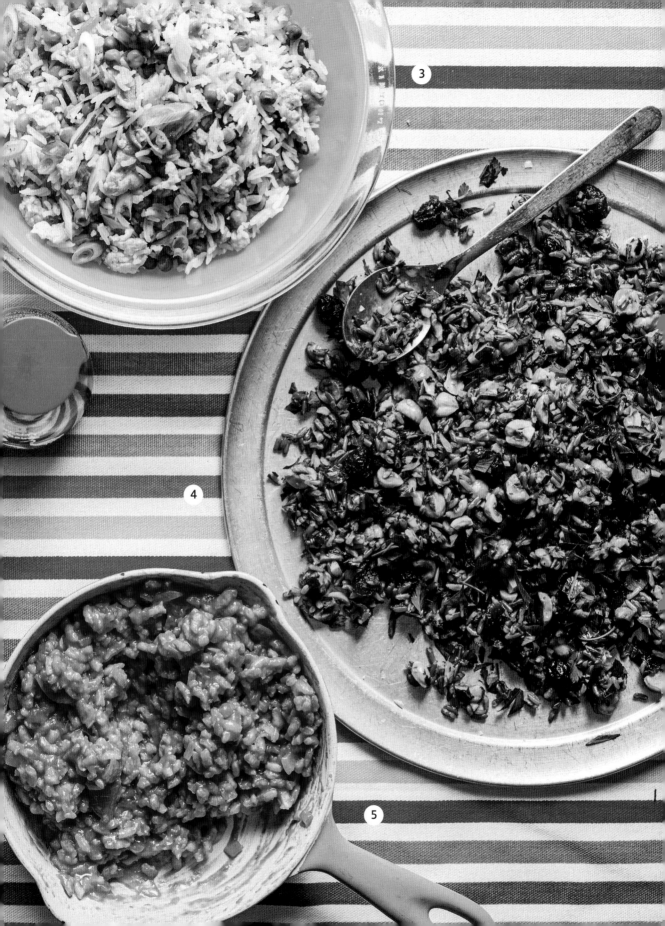

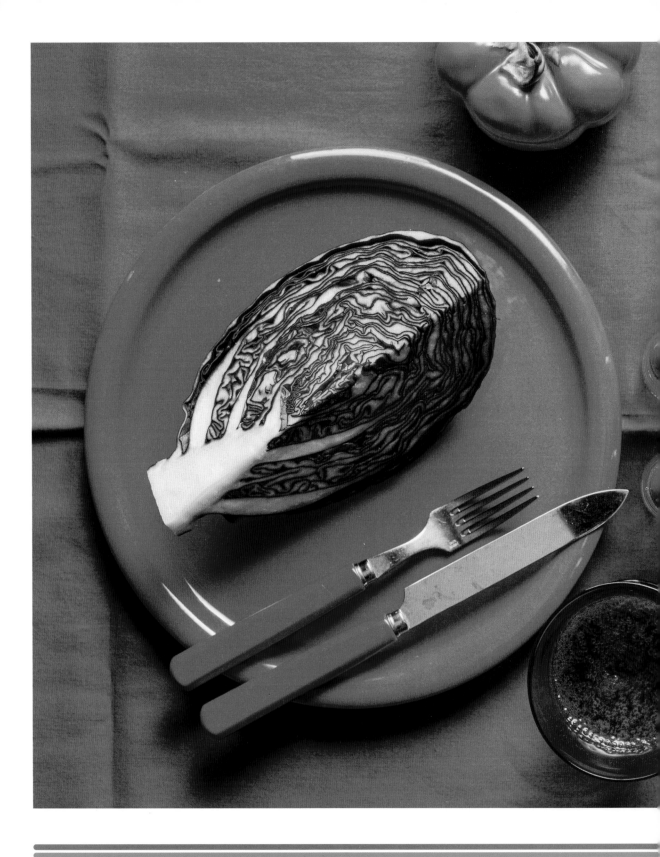

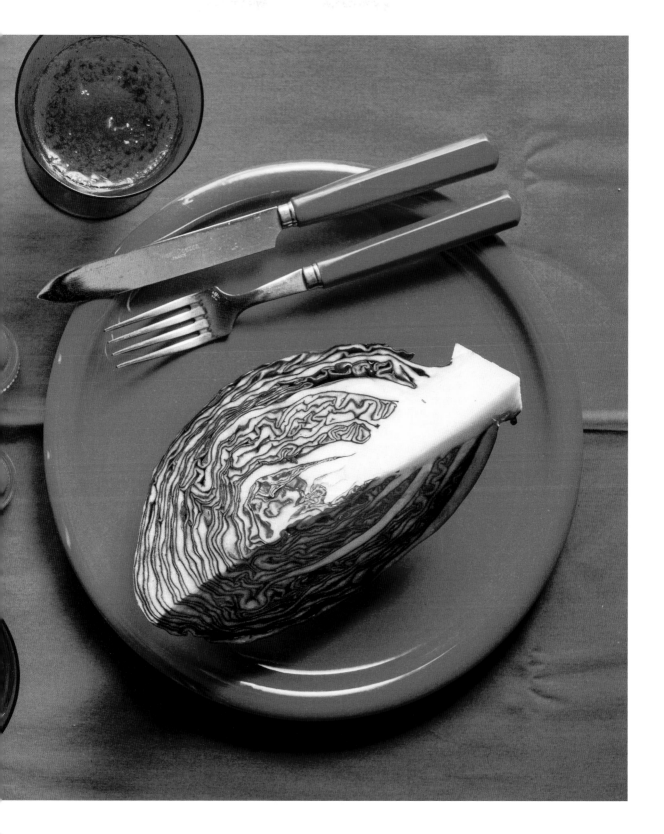

CUBBIES CLASSICS

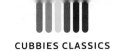
SAUCY BANGERS & MASH

Quite an involved-looking recipe for what is simply bangers and mash, but it's worth it for the gravy, we promise you. However, if you buy everything and decide to grill the sausages and open the Bisto, there's no judgement here. I confess to not being immediately sold on the addition of the apple, but like Paul behind the wheel of his tiny toy car, we'll never steer you wrong.

The slightly curried sauce makes this a little bit like a currywurst if you really squint your eyes, and that's simply no bad thing.

SERVES: 4
PREP: 15 minutes
COOK: 40 minutes
CALORIES: 496

1½ tablespoons cornflour
800g (1lb 12oz) potatoes
1 egg
1 knob of butter
8 good pork sausages
1 green apple, cored (no need to peel)
1 onion, peeled and sliced
2 cloves of garlic, crushed or grated
1 × 400g (14oz) tin of chopped tomatoes
1 teaspoon dried thyme
1½ teaspoons curry powder
1 teaspoon honey
½ teaspoon chilli flakes
1 beef stock cube, crumbled
salt and black pepper

In a small jug, mix the cornflour with 3 tablespoons of cold water and set aside.

Dice the potatoes (no need to peel) into 3cm (1¼ inch) chunks, then place in a large pan and cover with water. Bring to the boil, then simmer for 20–25 minutes until tender.

Remove the potatoes from the heat and drain, then put back into the pan to steam. Crack in the egg, add the butter and a pinch of salt and pepper, and mash to your liking.

Meanwhile, spray a large frying pan with a little oil and place over a medium heat. Add the sausages and cook for 10–15 minutes until browned, then remove from the pan and set aside.

Slice the apple and add to the frying pan, along with the onions and garlic. Cook for 5 minutes, stirring occasionally.

Add the chopped tomatoes, then fill the empty tin with 250ml (9fl oz) of water and pour that into the pan. Add the thyme, curry powder, honey and chilli flakes, then crumble over the stock cube and stir to mix.

Slice each of the cooked sausages into four and add to the sauce. Pour over the cornflour mix and stir well. Cook for 15–20 minutes, until thickened, then serve with the mash.

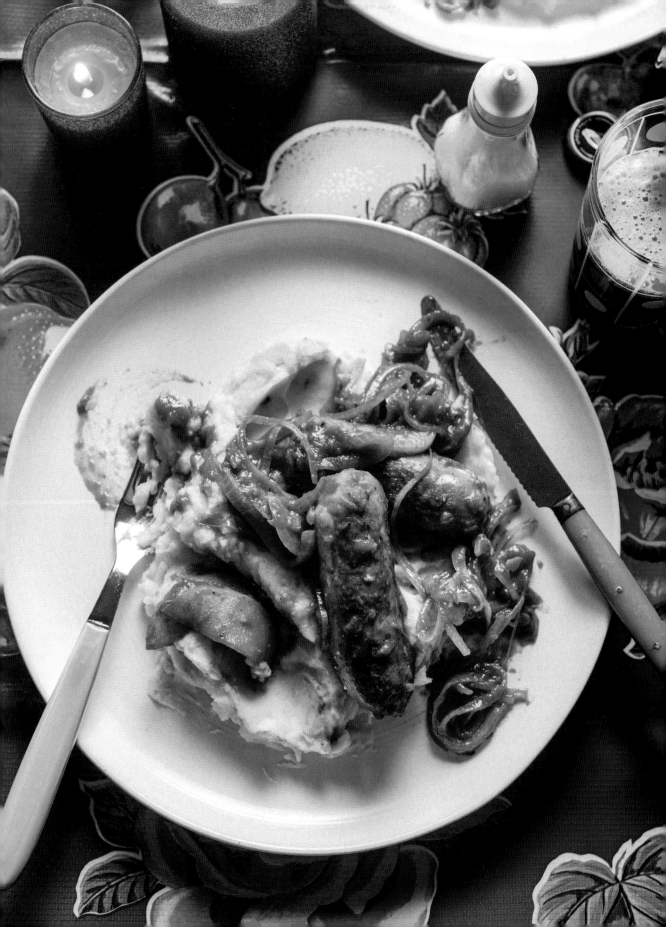

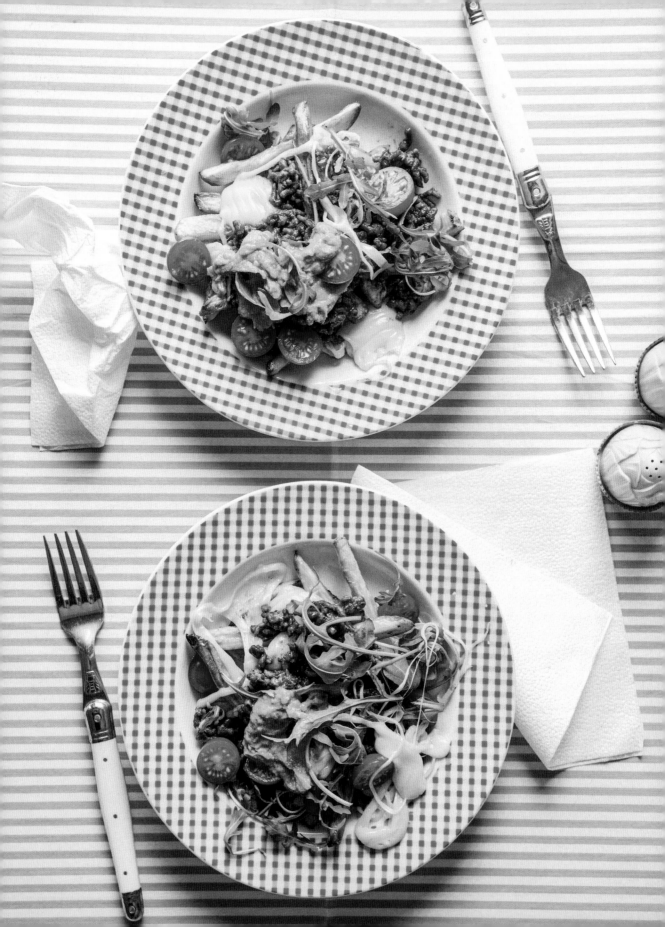

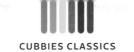
BEEF & CHEESE FRITTEN

This is a recent update to our recipe list, coming to us via a weekend in Hamburg where we sat under giant horse-chestnut trees in a lovely market and gorged ourselves on chips and mince. Well, I did – Paul had a salad because he thinks he's better than everyone else, but what can you do? Our host, a smile clad in lederhosen, tried to steer us into the restaurant but we ached to sit outside in the sun: a year of lockdown meant we were desperately short on vitamin D (not like us, admittedly) and it was taking forever to walk any distance with Paul's bandy legs.

We could see there were plenty of tables free, so we assured the waitress that we weren't vampires and were therefore quite content to be outside, and she dutifully showed us to our seats. A great meal was had, interrupted only by the real reason for recommending we took an inside seat becoming apparent: conkers falling to the ground from up high with a resounding crack. Naturally, being stoic, British and altogether too fat to move, we endured for as long as we could, moving only when an especially large conker dropped smartly, almost perfectly, straight off the top of Paul's head and into my cherry mimosa. You mustn't say we don't suffer for your recipes.

Either way, we can't pretend that this is anything more than gussied-up mince and chips. But then, dear reader, aren't we all?

SERVES: 4
PREP: 10 minutes
COOK: 45 minutes
CALORIES: 389

600g (1lb 5oz) potatoes
250g (9oz) lean beef mince
120g (4½oz) Cheddar cheese,
    grated
4 handfuls of rocket
16 cherry tomatoes, halved
4 tablespoons guacamole
salt

For the BBQ sauce

4 tablespoons tomato sauce
1 tablespoon brown sugar
1 tablespoon Worcestershire
    sauce
2 teaspoons cider vinegar
¼ teaspoon garlic granules
¼ teaspoon mustard powder

Chop the potatoes into chips, spray with a little oil, sprinkle with salt and cook to your liking in an air-fryer or in the oven.

Meanwhile, brown the mince in a frying pan over a medium-high heat.

In a bowl mix together the BBQ sauce ingredients, add to the pan, and cook until sticky.

Just before the chips are cooked, put the cheese into a microwave-safe bowl and heat on full power in the microwave for 15 seconds. Stir and repeat until nicely melted.

When the chips are cooked, divide between the plates and spoon over the melted cheese, then spoon over the beef.

Top with the rocket, cherry tomatoes and guacamole.

NOTE

No air-fryer? Spread the chips out on a non-stick baking tray and cook in the oven at 200°C fan/425°F/gas mark 7 for 30 minutes, turning halfway.

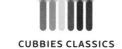
TURKEY CRUMBLE

Turkey crumble – have you ever heard of such a thing? Well, pop your jaw back up, it's really not as outrageous as the title may suggest: it's just a savoury, wonderful pleasure. Admittedly we wouldn't recommend serving it with custard, but you do you.

My nana – of the cheese pudding recipe mentioned earlier – did a mean crumble. Literally, she was mean with the filling: a thimble of apple sauce and a dandruff of crumble and that was your lot, but it was delicious. That's the old way of cooking though: not a lot, and served looking like something you'd see slid under a prison door, but wonderful. Mind, she did also used to pour enough salt to brine a fully-grown cow into her dinner, so perhaps we don't look to the past too reverentially if we want to live past forty.

Anyway: turkey crumble. Give it a go, let us know what you think, and send any cheques straight to our publishers.

SERVES: 4
PREP: 15 minutes
COOK: 1 hour
CALORIES: 450

400g (14oz) turkey mince
1 carrot, peeled and finely diced
1 onion, finely diced
2 cloves of garlic, crushed
1 chicken stock cube
150g (5½oz) spinach
60g (2¼oz) butter
100g (3½oz) plain flour
1 teaspoon dried oregano
½ teaspoon garlic granules
½ teaspoon salt
40g (1½oz) rolled oats
60g (2¼oz) reduced-fat mature
   Cheddar cheese, grated

Preheat the oven to 180°C fan/400°F/gas mark 6.

Spray a large frying pan with a little oil and place over a medium-high heat. Add the turkey mince, carrot, onion and garlic and cook until no pink meat remains.

Dissolve the stock cube in 300ml (10fl oz) of boiling water and add to the pan. Stir and simmer until thickened.

Add the spinach to the pan and cook until wilted.

Remove the mixture from the heat and set aside.

Meanwhile, in a bowl mix together the butter, flour, oregano, garlic granules, salt and rolled oats until it resembles crumble.

Tip the meat mixture into an ovenproof dish and cover with the crumble, then sprinkle over the Cheddar cheese.

Bake in the oven for 30 minutes, until golden.

NOTE

If freezing, do so before baking – once the filling is cool, cover the dish and freeze. Defrost thoroughly before cooking.

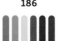

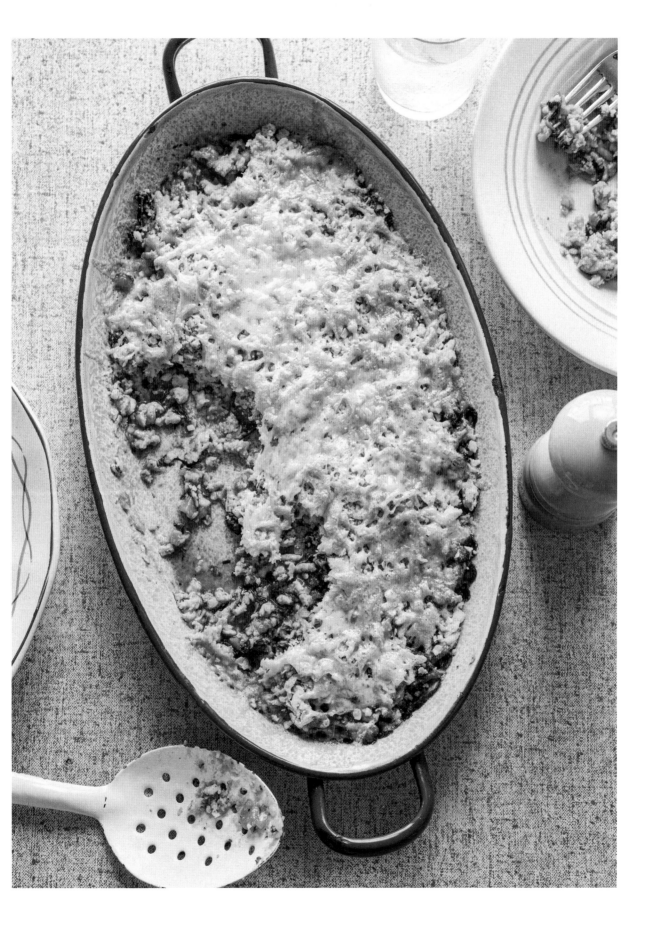

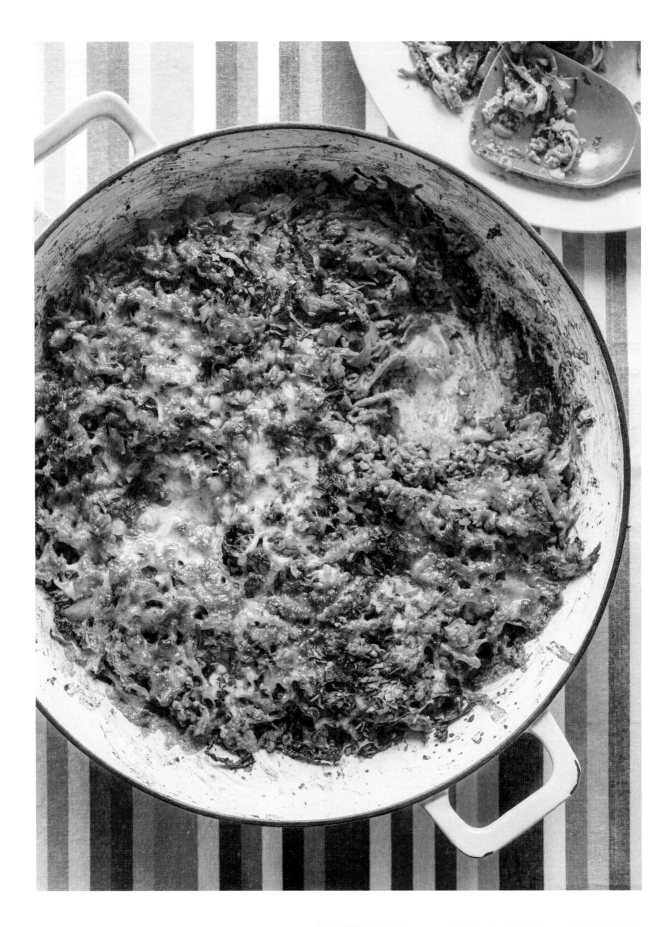

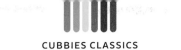
PROPER LAZY HUNGARIAN CABBAGE ROLLS

You know how occasionally you love the sound of something, make it and end up looking aghast at what the food gods have managed to turn your effort and labour into? That'll be this dish, we promise. Although our stylists have made it look gorgeous in the photo, we can almost guarantee yours will look like something growing on the side of a bin: it's the nature of the recipe. However, we can make a solemn vow of utter deliciousness: a tasty, simmering, cheese-topped wonder.

If you're not a fan of cabbage you may be reluctant, but rather like the You Fink Frank Wants Stew recipe on page 99, it's the flavour combination of this dish that really makes it work.

Oh, and we ought to say: this is very much a lazy, express version of cabbage rolls – if you have the time to take a look at the in-depth way of doing them, we encourage you to do so. It isn't hyperbole to say that cabbage rolls are easily one of our go-to dinners, and one day, they could be yours.

SERVES: 4
PREP: 15 minutes
COOK: 40 minutes
CALORIES: 364

1 onion, diced
500g (1lb 2oz) pork mince
1 tablespoon smoked paprika
1 tablespoon hot chilli powder
½ teaspoon garlic granules
2 teaspoons dried mixed herbs
2 teaspoons ground cumin
1 teaspoon ground coriander
1 tablespoon cider vinegar
100g (3½oz) low-fat soft cheese
125ml (4fl oz) passata
½ Savoy cabbage, thinly sliced
1 carrot, grated
80g (2¾oz) mozzarella cheese, grated
1 bunch of parsley, chopped

Preheat the oven to 180°C fan/400°F/gas mark 6.

Spray a large casserole dish with a little oil and place over a medium-high heat. Add the onion and cook for 5 minutes, until starting to turn golden.

Add the pork mince, paprika, chilli powder, garlic granules, mixed herbs, cumin, coriander and cider vinegar and stir. Cook for 5–10 minutes, until no pink meat remains.

Stir in the soft cheese and passata, then remove from the heat.

Add the cabbage and carrot to the pan and stir, then cover with the lid and bake in the oven for 45 minutes.

Remove from the oven, stir, and top with the cheese. Put back into the oven for a further 10–15 minutes (without the lid).

Set the oven grill to high. Place the dish under the hot grill for a few minutes, until the cheese is browned.

Remove from the oven, sprinkle over the parsley, and serve.

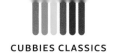
WE'VE BEEN AROUND THE WORLD AND WE WE WE — WE QUITE LIKE THIS (BISCUITS & SAUSAGE) GRAVY

You have no idea – none – the toll it has taken on me to try and top the pun of 'Nicely Spicy Easy Cheesy Yellow Butternut Linguine' from the last book. And, in the spirit of being honest, I don't think I will ever top it, even after spending hours awake in bed desperately trying.

'Biscuits and gravy' is one of those meals that looks like someone's already had a bash at digesting it, but it tastes so, so good. The biscuits are not the biscuits you may expect as a confirmed dieter, but rather what we know as scones. We have tipped a wink to an old blog favourite and made 'scones' from cottage cheese and mashed potatoes – they're not the abomination that we expected and we genuinely implore you to give them a go!

SERVES: 4
PREP: 15 minutes
COOK: 25 minutes
CALORIES: 332

2 eggs
300g (10½oz) fat-free cottage cheese
100g (3½oz) instant mash
30g (1oz) mature Cheddar cheese, grated
3 tablespoons chopped chives
2 cloves of garlic, crushed
140g (5oz) low-fat sausages
2 tablespoons plain flour
300ml (10fl oz) milk
salt and black pepper

NOTES

The scone recipe here is one we used years ago on the blog but it still holds up. If you can't be a*sed, though, a plain scone, an English muffin or any bun will do the trick.

Preheat the oven to 190°C fan/425°F/gas mark 7 and line a baking tray with greaseproof paper.

Blend together the eggs and cottage cheese (ideally with a stick blender).

Add the instant mash, cheese, chives and garlic and mix until it forms a dough-like consistency (add a little more water if too dry or a bit more mash if too wet).

Shape into 6 balls and squash into a rough scone shape. Bake in the oven for 25 minutes, then remove from the oven and allow to cool.

Meanwhile, score the sausages with a knife (careful) and peel away the skin to get to the good meaty stuff. Discard the skins and roughly chop the sausage meat.

Place a frying pan over a medium heat and spray with a little oil. Add the sausage meat to the frying pan and cook for 5–6 minutes, until nicely browned, breaking it up with a wooden spoon as you go (ideally you want it to resemble mince, but don't worry if the chunks look a bit bigger – that's fine).

Add the flour to the pan and stir. Gradually add the milk and stir constantly, while gently bringing the mix to the boil. Reduce the heat to medium-low and simmer for another 2 minutes, stirring constantly. Season with salt and pepper to your liking.

Split the scones in half and place on the plates (3 halves each). Pour over the sausage gravy.

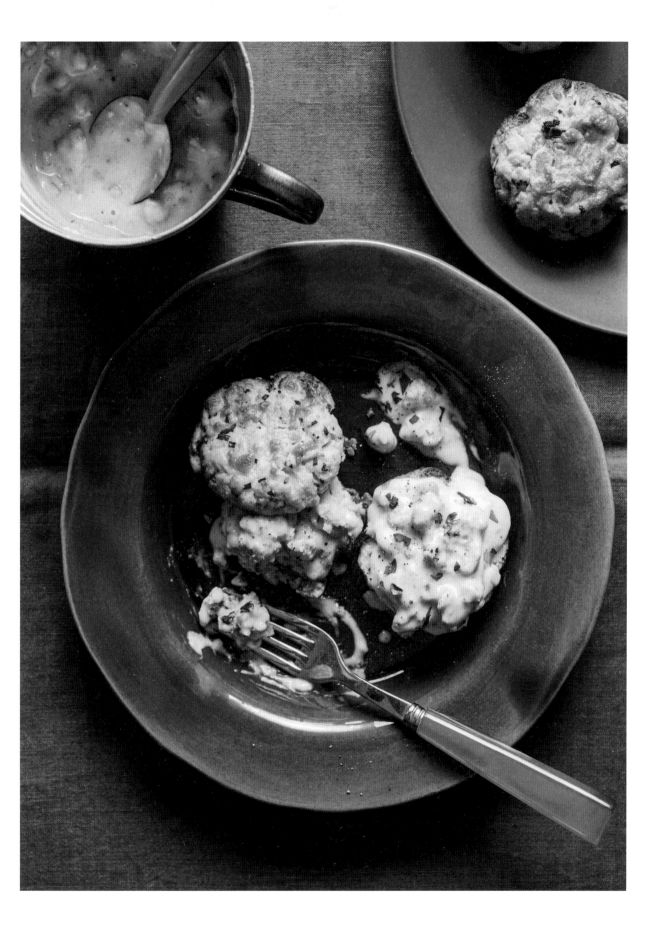

BRINED PORK CHOPS

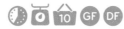

For at least thirty-five years of our adult lives we had both been 'enjoying' pork chops that were grey, tough and didn't exactly burst with flavour. That suited Paul, a man whose idea of adventure is eating an after-eight at half seven, but I always longed for much more.

It wasn't until last year that a very good friend introduced me to the art of brining a pork chop and changed my life. He introduced me to all sorts of other things too, but I'm saving that for our tell-all autobiography when Paul and I are at least sixty. Working title: 'Hard to Swallow', happy for the bidding rights to begin at any time.

As is utterly typical with me, I immediately forgot everything he taught me the second I got back home and was too proud to ask for further instruction. Remembering the key ingredients at least, I cobbled together the recipe below – feel free to experiment with your own tweaks. Paul adores these, as I adore him.

SERVES: 4
PREP: 10 minutes
COOK: 40 minutes
MARINATING: 1 hour
CALORIES: 624

50g (1¾oz) brown sugar
50g (1¾oz) salt
juice of 2 limes
1 × 340g (12oz) jar of jalapeños, chopped finely, keeping the liquid
8 fat pork chops

Put the sugar, salt, lime juice and jalapenos into a pan with 500ml (18fl oz) water and bring to the boil. Stir until all the sugar and salt has dissolved, then leave to cool.

Once the brine has cooled, pack your pork chops into a Pyrex dish and pour the brine over, making sure everything is covered.

Cover with foil and allow to marinate for an hour or longer in the fridge.

To cook the chops, simply blot them dry, then place under the grill, turning them once, until cooked through.

NOTES

We have to confess – there's absolutely no rhyme or reason to this brine – we just go with the flavours we know we like.

We serve these with chips for a good simple dinner – no fanciness here!

One important thing: do not add the pork to the brine until the brine has cooled right down – you don't want the pork to start cooking until it is under the grill.

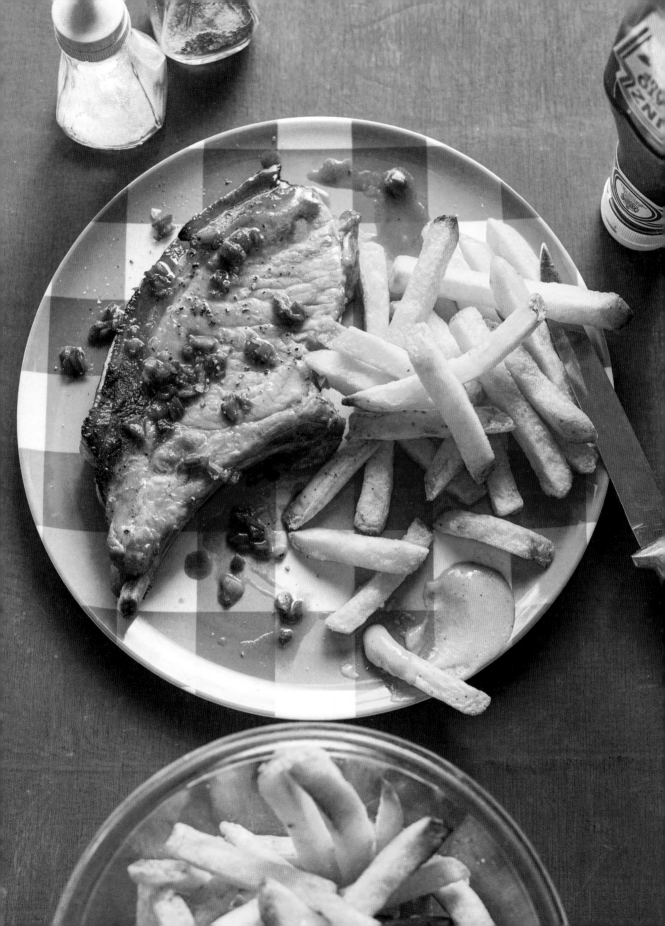

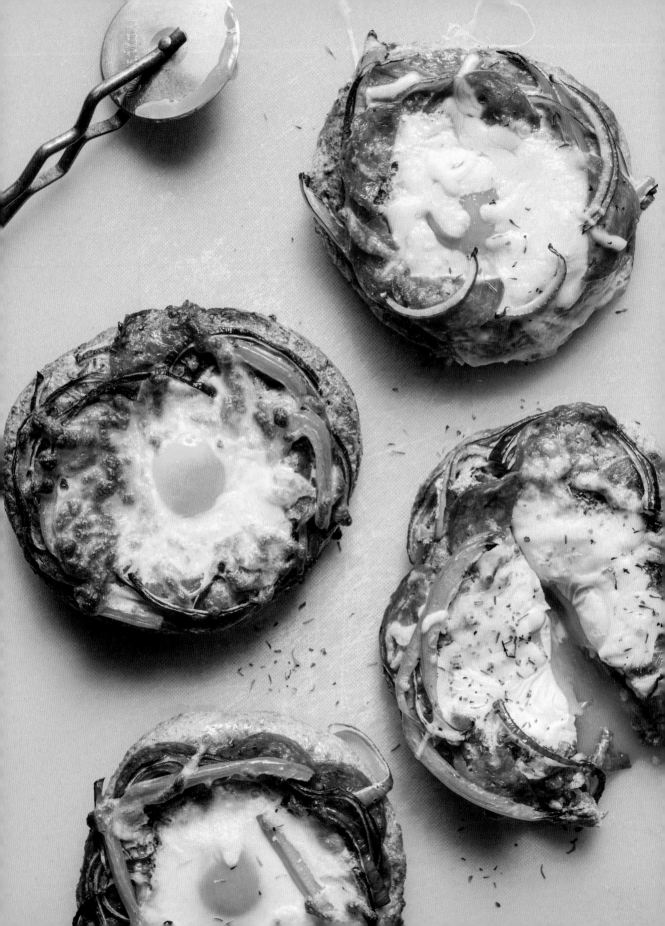

LITTLE BRUNCHY PIZZAS

Readers of the previous book will remember my utter disgust at Paul's use of the words 'lil' and 'fam', when he's about as street as a beige carpet. Clearly my tittylipping didn't sink in, as he's back to test us all with 'brunchy'. I have asked for clarification as to whether that is a riff on crunchy or simply that these little pizzas are a good bridge between breakfast and lunch, but the answer isn't forthcoming. A man of secrets.

We know this goes without saying, but please do not be locked to the topping we suggest. You can put all sorts on to these, but we rather like the somewhat accusatory eyeball look you get from the eggs cracked into the middle.

SERVES: 4
PREP: 1 hour 30 minutes (including proving time)
COOK: 20 minutes
CALORIES: 434

2 teaspoons sugar
1 × 7g sachet fast-action dried yeast
5 eggs
200g (7oz) wholewheat flour
½ teaspoon salt
1 tablespoon olive oil
3 tablespoons passata
1 teaspoon dried mixed herbs
50g (1¾oz) pepperoni slices, cut in half
1 red onion, sliced
1 red pepper, deseeded and sliced
75g (2¾oz) grated mozzarella cheese
30g (1oz) parsley, chopped

First, make the dough by whisking together the sugar, yeast and 1 egg with 250ml (9fl oz) of warm water in a medium bowl. Leave the mixture in a warm place for 10–15 minutes, to activate the yeast.

Add a third of the flour to the bowl, along with the salt and olive oil, and mix until well combined. Add the remaining flour to the mix and knead until nicely elastic.

Transfer the dough to a large bowl sprayed with a little oil, cover with cling film and leave to rise for 1 hour.

Preheat the oven to 200°Cfan/425°F/gas mark 7.

Gently knead the dough, then divide it into 4 pieces and roll each one into a ball. Place them on a baking sheet lined with greaseproof paper. Gently push your thumb into the middle of each ball to make a well, forming a sort of doughnut shape (but don't press too deeply!).

Spread the passata over each of the balls, including in the well, and sprinkle over the mixed herbs. Arrange the pepperoni, onions and peppers around the edge of each pizza.

Crack an egg into each of the wells and sprinkle over the mozzarella. Scatter over the parsley and bake in the oven for 15–20 minutes, until browned.

Serve with a salad.

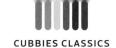
LAZY ROAST DINNER

 GF DF

We adore a Sunday dinner here at Chubby Towers, and I will cheerfully tell anyone what an expert Paul is at making a perfectly timed, gloriously tasty spread with a minimum of fuss. To give you some idea of his talents, know this: the man managed to deliver a roast dinner every second Sunday when all we had was a one-ring induction hob and an oven. He's a treasure!

However, Paul also works terrifically hard, and sometimes Sunday needs to be a day of sitting on his tush watching TV, sitting on his tush looking at his phone or lying on his back in bed, asleep. On those rare occasions when Action Jackson needs a rest, we'll often pull together this zippy little roast instead and let the oven do most of the hard work. It's not quite as extravagant as a full roast dinner, but it's still a bloody wonder. Enjoy!

SERVES: 4
PREP: 10 minutes
COOK: 1 hour 30 minutes
CALORIES: 500

400g (14oz) potatoes
2 onions
1 head of broccoli, cut into florets
½ teaspoon dried mixed herbs
½ teaspoon salt
¼ teaspoon black pepper
100ml (3½fl oz) white wine
1 tablespoon olive oil
3 cloves of garlic, crushed or grated
½ teaspoon onion granules
½ teaspoon dried thyme
½ teaspoon dried rosemary
1 whole chicken

Preheat the oven to 180°C fan/400°F/gas mark 6.

Dice the potatoes into bite-size chunks (no need to peel). Peel and slice the onions.

Spray a large casserole dish with a little oil and arrange the potatoes, onions and broccoli over the base. Add the mixed herbs, salt and pepper and toss to combine, then pour the wine into the bottom of the dish (but not over the potatoes).

In a small bowl mix together the olive oil, garlic, onion granules, dried thyme, dried rosemary and a pinch of salt and pepper.

Pat the chicken dry and gently brush over the olive oil mix. Put the chicken on top of the potatoes and cover with the lid. Roast in the oven for 1 hour. After an hour, remove the lid and roast for another 30 minutes.

Remove from the oven and leave to rest for 10 minutes, then carve and serve.

NOTE

A good ovenproof casserole dish is what you need here – we've got a Le Creuset that does the job perfectly, but cheaper alternatives exist and work just as well.

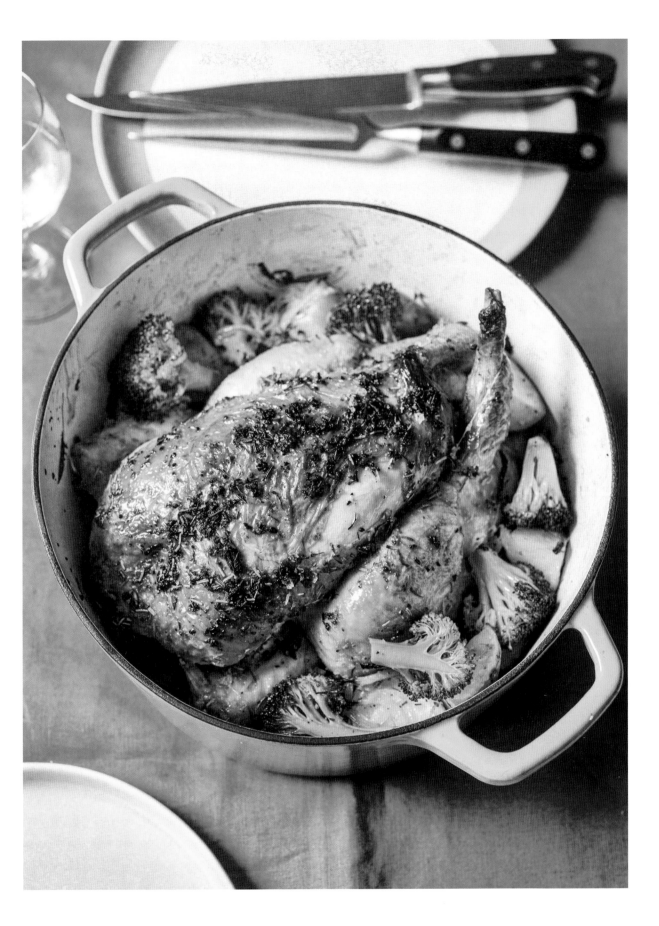

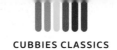
STRAWBERRY PORK LOIN

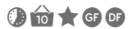

There's something about a pork loin that we both love – an undeniable quality that just speaks to us. We can't think for one moment why handling a ten-inch length of thick pork brings us such joy. However, it does explain why Paul was asked to leave the meat aisle in Waitrose that time.

Strawberry and pork might seem like one of those pairings that make your lips go all cats-bum, but should you take a moment to think about it, it's nothing more dramatic than a plum sauce, is it? Sticky and sweet. To be fair, if we had used plums, I'd have probably ended up with a hernia from trying to hold back all the puns in the world.

SERVES: 4
PREP: 10 minutes
COOK: 2 hours 5 minutes
CALORIES: 432

1 pork tenderloin (1kg)
8 slices of bacon
2 cloves of garlic, finely chopped
    or crushed
125ml (4fl oz) balsamic vinegar
300g (10½oz) ripe strawberries,
    sliced
1 big bag of rocket or other green
    leaf

Preheat the oven to 200°C fan/425°F/gas mark 7.

Wrap the tenderloin in bacon – secure it with cocktail sticks if you like – and put it into a small roasting tin. Cook it in the oven for around 30 minutes, then take it out, turn it over, and pop it back in for another 30 minutes.

Spray a large frying pan with oil and put it on a low heat. Add the garlic and fry it very gently until golden. Add the balsamic vinegar and half the strawberries. Bring to the boil, then reduce to a low simmer for about 10 minutes.

Once your pork is done, glaze it with a few spoonfuls of the strawberry balsamic and whack it under the grill for a couple of minutes.

Meanwhile, throw the rest of the sliced strawberries into the pan to get them sticky and to give a different texture for you to chew on.

Serve the pork sliced thickly, and the sauce drizzled over, with the rocket – nice and simple.

NOTE

Now listen here: this pork goes really, really well with the emotional support potatoes from book one – who knew that pork and potato would pair so well?

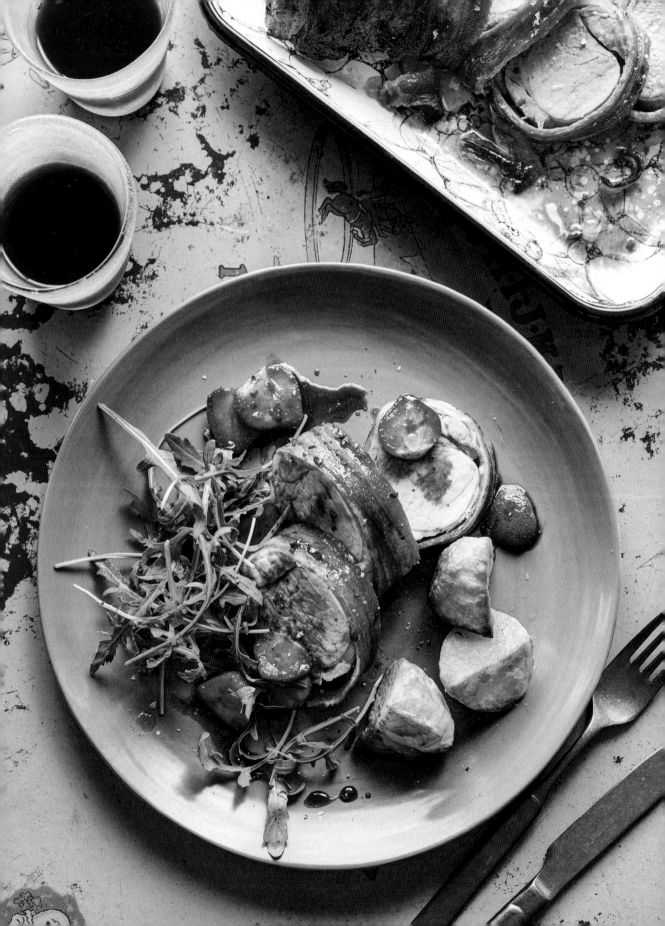

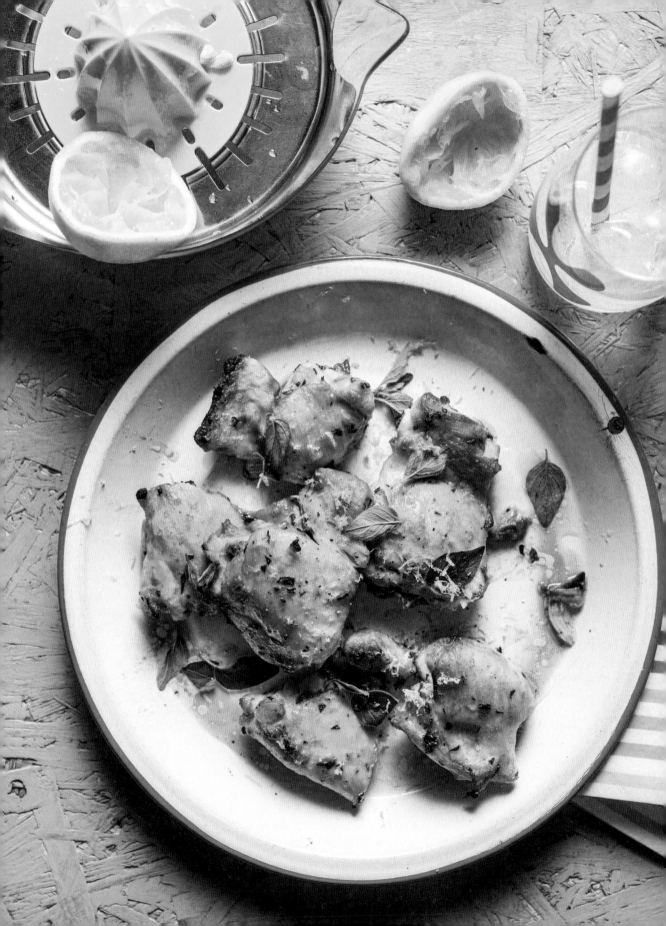

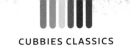
LEMON & OREGANO CHICKEN

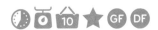

This recipe is a blog classic that we usually throw on the BBQ, but in the interests of ease we have replaced the thrilling experience with something you can do in the kitchen. Plus, we're a mite sensitive about open flames in the garden these days.

You know it's funny what you get used to, though. While our insurers (who were excellent) set about rebuilding our house, we were holed up in a hotel room for the best part of a year with barely enough room to swing a cat. With most of our possessions gone or in storage, we had quite the epiphany (one normally reserved for gap-yaaaah folks) that we had altogether too many things and vowed to have a cull when we returned to Chubby Towers.

Luckily, that moment was soon dashed the second we returned and realised we had an excuse to buy shiny new things, and now the house is fit to burst once more. We tried, though. Tell you what, mind, when I woke to the sight of the house merrily on fire, my only thought? Save Paul.

Mainly because I didn't want to have to take over cooking the recipes, admittedly, but again, the thought was there.

SERVES: 4
PREP: 35 minutes
COOK: 30 minutes
CALORIES: 227

zest of 1 lemon
120ml (4fl oz) lemon juice
2 tablespoons olive oil
2 tablespoons fresh oregano, chopped
a few fresh oregano sprigs
6–8 skinless, boneless chicken thighs

Combine the lemon zest and juice, oil and oregano together, rub over the chicken thighs, and leave to marinate for 30 minutes.

Preheat the oven to 220°C fan/475°F/gas mark 9.

Cook for 30 minutes until the juices run clear and the chicken is cooked.

Garnish with oregano leaves before serving.

NOTE

To cook this under a hot grill, make sure to turn the chicken regularly and make sure it's cooked through! Of course, if you want you can cook it over a hot barbecue – just cook until the juices run clear and the chicken is cooked.

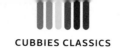
LEVINSON-~~GOULD'S~~ OSSO BUCO

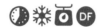

The perfect dinner to serve to colleagues over a dinner party, this osso buco is full of flavour, and although we have swapped out the traditional veal for beef here to avoid any angry letters, should you be that way inclined, you know what to do. However, we don't feel it loses anything for using beef, so please don't feel pressured. Paul once made this for me in the early stages of our relationship when I had finally broken down and bought myself a plasma TV. I was reticent at first – I couldn't prove it but I thought he might be trying to poison me – but I'm glad I gave it a chance. In fact, you could say … that one night, he made everything all right …

You know what the best part of that intro is? Most of you will probably assume I've had some kind of breakdown, but those who get it will enjoy it ever so. I'll be here all night, try the veal! Or swap it for beef, we don't care.

SERVES: 4
PREP: 10 minutes
COOK: 1 hour 45 minutes
CALORIES: 484

4 bacon medallions, diced
1 tablespoon flour
800g (1lb 12oz) diced beef
1 onion, finely diced
1 carrot, finely diced
2 celery stalks, finely diced
6 cloves of garlic, 4 finely diced,
    2 crushed
1 teaspoon dried thyme
250ml (9fl oz) white wine
500ml (18fl oz) chicken stock
1 × 400g (14oz) tin of chopped
    tomatoes
2 tablespoons finely diced fresh
    parsley
zest of ½ lemon

Preheat the oven to 170°C fan/375°F/gas mark 5.

Spray an ovenproof pan or casserole dish with a little oil and place over a medium-high heat.

Add the diced bacon and cook for 4–5 minutes, until crisp, then scoop on to a plate and set aside. Spray the pan with a bit more oil.

Sprinkle the flour over the beef along with a pinch of salt and pepper and add to the pan. Cook until the beef is browned, then remove from the pan and set aside.

Add the onion, carrot and celery and cook for about 5 minutes, until the onions are translucent. Add the diced garlic and thyme and stir, then cook for another 10 minutes.

Put the beef and bacon back into the pan and add the wine to deglaze, then add the stock and the chopped tomatoes. Bring everything to a simmer, cover with a lid, and cook in the oven for 1 hour 15 minutes.

Meanwhile, mix together the parsley, crushed garlic and lemon zest and put to one side.

Serve the beef with the parsley mix on top.

NOTE

This is traditionally served with polenta, but we love it with mash (which is much less faff).

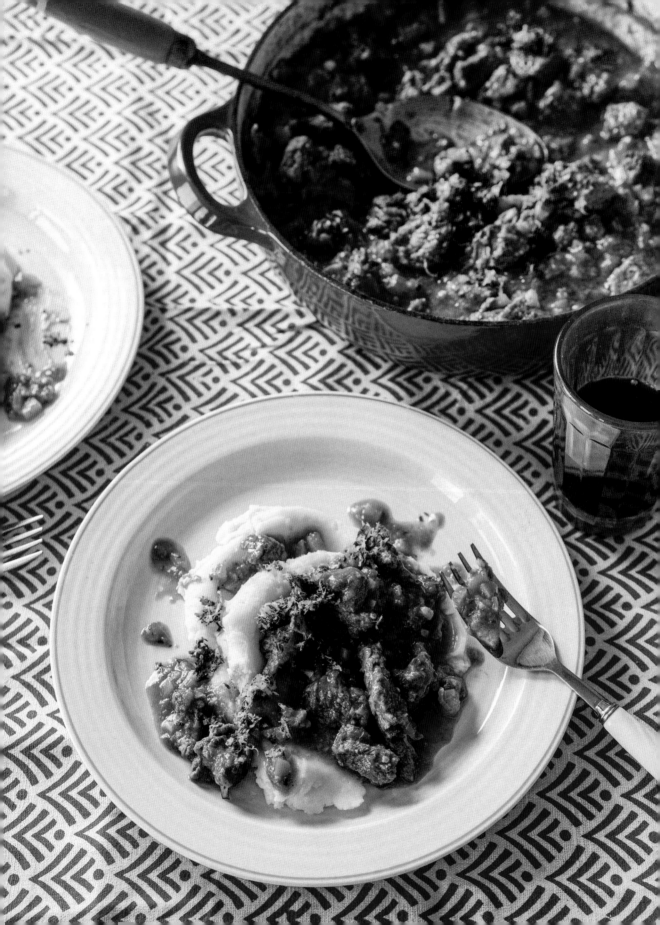

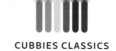
WHY AYE PIE

We aren't going to be drawn into what constitutes a pie: we all know the real answer is meat fully encased in pastry. We get it. This is a stew with a fancy hat, but sometimes it's a-OK to just roll with it, or indeed, have a roll with it, because that'll be handy for mopping up the gravy. See the notes, though.

Perhaps you're thinking that we only included this because we came up with 'why aye pie' and worked backwards to put Newcastle Brown Ale in. Yup. But in our defence, we've been making this beef pie for an age and only added the crunchy filo top to save on calories. You could forgo the top altogether (never!) and serve with mash if you wanted!

The smallest plea, while Newcastle is in our minds: come and visit! People who have never seen Newcastle seem to assume we all wander around with soot on our faces punching horses, and we simply don't. It's a city full of beautiful architecture, amazing food, lovely people and transformative views, plus, if you're lucky, you might bump into us waddling about looking lost and confused.

SERVES: 4
PREP: 10 minutes
COOK: 30 minutes
CALORIES: 324

500g (1lb 2oz) diced beef
1 large carrot, peeled and chopped
1 onion, chopped
2 cloves of garlic, crushed
1 tablespoon tomato purée
1 tablespoon Worcestershire sauce
1 tablespoon flour
½ beef stock cube
100ml (3½fl oz) Newcastle Brown Ale
¼ teaspoon dried thyme
¼ teaspoon dried rosemary
½ teaspoon salt
¼ teaspoon black pepper
4 filo pastry sheets
1 egg, beaten

Preheat the oven to 220° fan/475°F/gas mark 9.

Spray a large frying pan with a little oil and place over a medium-high heat. Add the beef and cook for 5–6 minutes, until browned all over, then remove to a plate and set aside.

Add the carrots and onion to the pan and cook for 5 minutes, until softened. Add the garlic, tomato purée and Worcestershire sauce and cook for another minute.

Add the flour and crumble in the stock cube, stir well until everything is mixed up, then add the brown ale and cook until the mix starts to thicken a bit.

Put the beef back into the pan along with the thyme, rosemary, salt and pepper, stir, then remove from the heat.

Tip the meat into an ovenproof dish.

Unroll the pastry sheets and brush with the beaten egg. Cut each sheet in half, then scrunch each one into a ball and place on top of the beef.

Bake in the oven for 15 minutes.

NOTES

Any ale will do, but of course Broon is best.

If freezing, do it before baking.

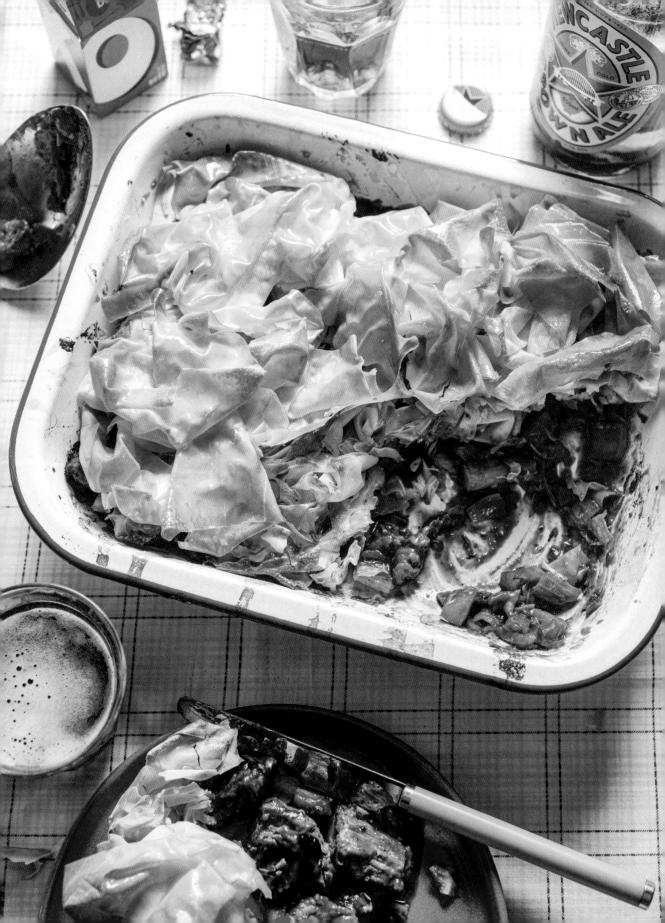

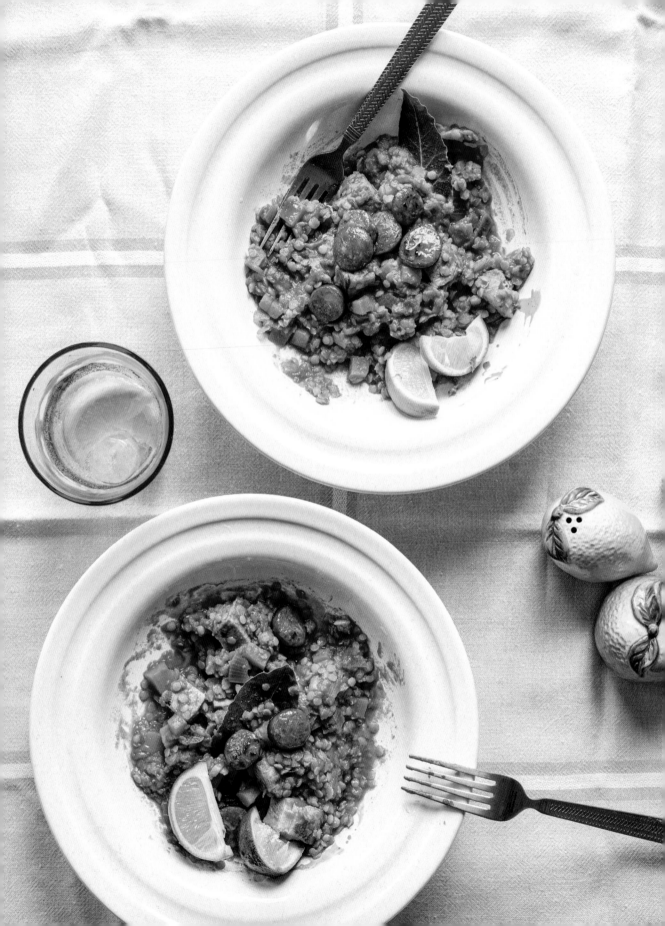

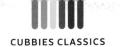
'OWT WITH A PULSE PORK

This recipe arrives with you via my good friend Paul Susan Hawkins, who has diva-demanded that his name is in the recipe introduction this time. Paul, 41, is a perfect example of why, if you're sat reading these recipes and feel unsure of your cooking ability, you must dash into the kitchen to get cooking without delay. During the various lockdowns of 2020, Paul, forever looking for a reason to shout at things, taught himself how to cook.

It's been like watching a blossoming flower. Recipes have been tinkered with, own spins have been added and confidence has come shining through. For all I tease, it's been lovely to see (and eat). He's very proud of this recipe, as we are of him.

There, that should get me twenty minutes of quiet.

SERVES: 4
PREP: 10 minutes
COOK: 1 hour 30 minutes
CALORIES: 500

4 pork loin steaks
1 red onion, chopped
1 large celery stalk, chopped
2 large carrots, peeled and chopped
2 cloves of garlic (see notes)
1 tablespoon smoked paprika
1 × 400g (14oz) tin of good chopped tomatoes
500ml (18fl oz) chicken stock
180g (6oz) dried red lentils
zest and juice of ½ lime
2 bay leaves
50g (1¾oz) chorizo picante
salt and black pepper

Over a medium heat, fry your pork loins in a good cast-iron pot until they have some colour – if you're not a heathen who cuts the fat off, make sure you push the fat down until it crisps a little – once coloured on both sides, cut into chunks and set aside.

Throw the onion, celery and carrot into the pan and soften over a medium heat, making sure to stir so nothing catches. Add the garlic and mix it through the vegetables for a minute or two, then add the paprika and do the same.

Add the tomatoes, stock, chopped pork, lentils, lime zest and bay leaves and give everything a good stir, adding a pinch of salt and pepper to taste. Bring to a simmer, then lower the heat so it can hurble-burble for about 25 minutes.

Towards the end of the 25 minutes, skin your chorizo (madam!) and chop into thick discs.

In a dry frying pan, fry the chorizo on each side so it gets a good deep crust, then remove and slice into quarters, keeping the oil in the pan.

Check your lentils – you want them softened but not too mushy, so if there's too much liquid, whack the heat up for 5 minutes to thicken.

Add the chorizo, the chorizo oil and the lime juice, then stir – try to fish the bay leaves out if you spot them. Taste, and add some salt if needed.

NOTES

For the garlic: a rare occasion where you're better off chopping it finely or using a press rather than grating, as you want a more mellow taste.

This makes enough for 4 generous portions, so you could easily save a bit for lunch the next day.

We used red lentils, but green lentils do just as well.

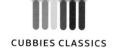
PORK & CHERRY PINWHEELS

These pork and cherry pinwheels are a fantastic evening meal and look both inviting and fancy when you come to serve them up. It's the type of dish that you might enjoy on a summer's evening outside in the garden, though not if you are us: we are forever locked in some sort of mild dispute with at least one set of neighbours wherever we have lived, and thus being outside is a strained affair. Now, you may think of the saying 'If you smell muck everywhere you go, look at your own shoes', and perhaps you would be right, but you have to understand we are delightful to live alongside. Imagine having two overweight men barrelling around their kitchen, forgetting to put the blinds down or their clothes on, shrieking and yelling and causing a scene. You'd dash out of bed every morning like your a*se was on fire, wouldn't you?

I jest. Perhaps if you have problematic neighbours, though, you could make this deliciously simple supper and win them over?

SERVES: 4
PREP: 15 minutes
COOK: 30 minutes
CALORIES: 390

750g (1lb 10oz) pork tenderloin
3 tablespoons cherry jam
4 slices of prosciutto
80g (3oz) frozen spinach, thawed
    and all liquid squeezed out
40g (1½oz) Wensleydale cheese
    with cranberries, crumbled
1 tablespoon butter
2 cloves of garlic, crushed
    or grated
1 teaspoon fresh thyme leaves
125ml (4fl oz) red wine
1 teaspoon balsamic vinegar

Preheat the oven to 220°C fan/475°F/gas mark 9.

Butterfly the pork and spread with 2 tablespoons of the cherry jam, then layer with the prosciutto, spinach and Wensleydale cheese.

Roll the pork lengthways and secure with string or cocktail sticks.

Spray a large ovenproof roasting dish with a little oil and place over a medium-high heat. Add the pork and cook for 1 minute on each side.

Transfer the dish to the oven and roast for 20 minutes, then remove from the oven, wrap the pork in foil and leave to rest.

Put the roasting dish back on the hob and add the butter, garlic and thyme. Stir constantly until the butter has melted.

Add the wine and balsamic vinegar, and simmer for a few minutes. Stir in the remaining cherry jam, then remove from the heat.

Unwrap the pork, cut into 2cm (¾ inch) slices, and drizzle over the sauce to serve.

NOTES

Apricot jam is also a belter in this!

Use any cheese you like. Blue cheese is a great alternative if you swing that way.

If you don't have a suitable roasting dish that will go on the stovetop, you can cook the pork in a large frying pan and then transfer it to a roasting tin.

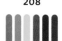

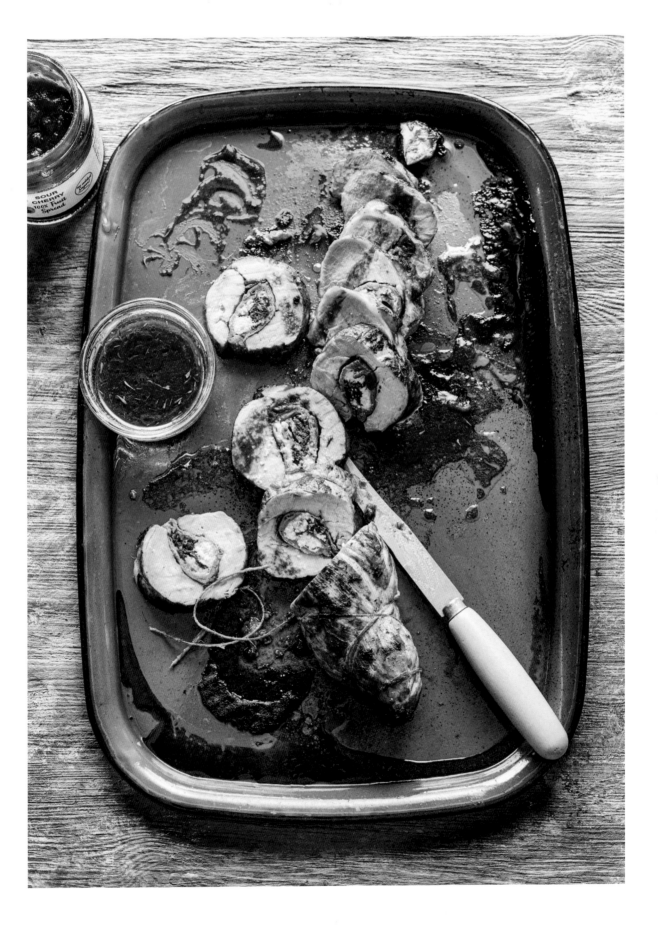

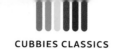
PAN HAGGERTY'S PAN HAGGERTY

DCI Kenneth Sexington hadn't always had a permanent frown, of course, and it would be foolish to think otherwise. He hadn't even always been a Sexington. As a child he had been described as a walking smile who had lit up every room he entered. This was never more true than the time he carried his mother's birthday cake to the dining table, his eyelashes sizzling gently from the heat of the sixty joke-shop candles wobbling on the top. He had spent the afternoon with his face in his mother's recipe book, following her spidery handwriting to make the perfect chocolate cake. How she had beamed as they set the cake down and, as Kenneth's family burst into a rousing rendition of 'Happy Birthday' that could be heard four streets over, she had set about trying to blow the candles out.

The verdict delivered at the inquest afterwards would record that Pandora Haggerty, 60 (just), died from a massive heart attack brought on by four minutes of attempting to extinguish the candles. Kenneth would never smile again.

This recipe belonged to his mother, and while she is no longer around to dish it up for her loved ones, it is hoped that you find this potatoey, cheesy, oniony wonder a comfort indeed.

SERVES: 4
PREP: 10 minutes
COOK: 40 minutes
CALORIES: 333

600g (1lb 5oz) potatoes
1 onion
1 tablespoon butter
3 bacon medallions, chopped
1 large leek, sliced
70g (2½oz) mature Cheddar
    cheese, grated
1 teaspoon dried parsley
1 teaspoon garlic granules
a handful of chives, sliced

NOTES

Trust me, the butter makes all the difference, but a spray of oil will be fine if you need to.

Compressing the layers makes it nice and crispy and in my opinion is worth the effort, but for a cheat's version you can simply cook the lot on the hob for 30 minutes.

Preheat the oven to 200°C fan/425°F/gas mark 7.

Thinly slice the potatoes and onion, and set aside.

Put the butter into a large frying pan and place over a medium heat. Add the bacon and leeks and cook until softened, then remove to a plate.

Return the pan to the heat and spray with a little oil. Spread a layer of the sliced potatoes in the bottom of the pan, then add the onions, bacon and leeks, followed by half the cheese and the parsley. Top with another layer of potatoes and the remaining cheese.

Spray the top of the potatoes with a bit more oil, then cover the pan with a lid (or tin foil) and cook for 15 minutes.

Remove the lid and place a sheet of greaseproof paper on top. Gently press down with a clean plate to help compact the layers. Remove the plate but keep the paper in the pan and put the lid back on top.

Put the pan into the oven and cook for 15 minutes, then compress again (careful now, it'll be hot) and cook for another 15 minutes.

Gently tip on to a chopping board and slice into wedges. Sprinkle over the chives.

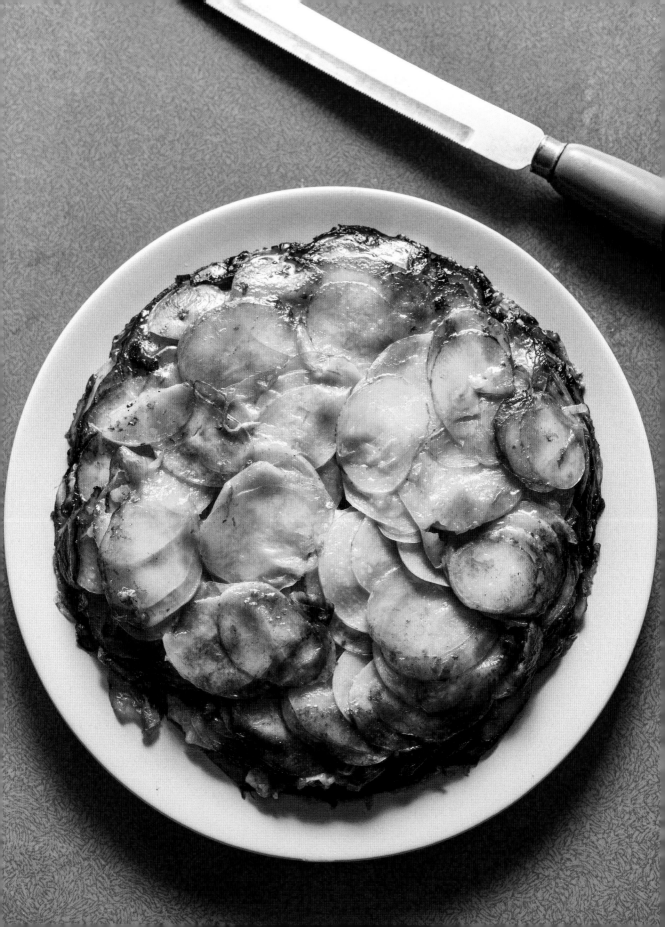

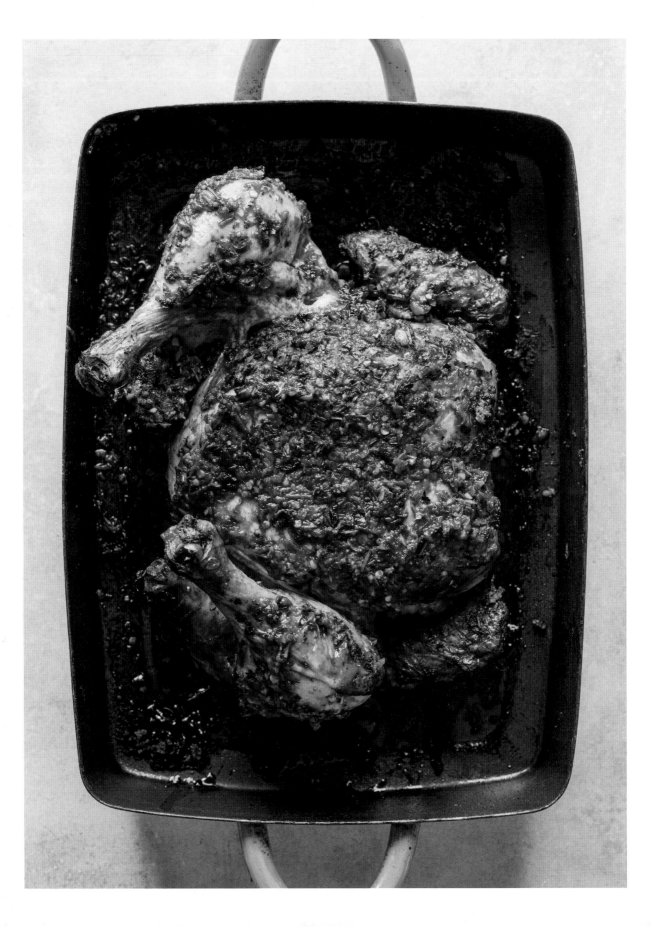

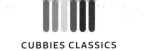
PERI-PERI SPATCHCOCKED CHICKEN

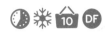

We're going to keep this short because we're going technical, baby – but just know this. If you're the sort of person who describes a particular chicken retailer as in any way cheeky, you'll be the first ones booted out of our utopia. It's really that simple, Susan.

But, for what it's worth, this is BLOODY DELICIOUS.

SERVES: 4
PREP: 15 minutes
COOK: 1 hour 15 minutes
CALORIES: 412

6 red chillies
1 whole chicken
2 tomatoes
5 cloves of garlic
juice of 1 lemon
2 tablespoons malt vinegar
20g (¾oz) fresh flat-leaf parsley
1 teaspoon smoked paprika
1 teaspoon dried oregano
1 teaspoon sugar
2 teaspoons salt

Preheat the grill to high. Grill the chillies for 7–8 minutes, until charred, then set aside.

Turn the chicken over so the breasts are face down on the chopping board. Using a good pair of scissors, cut away at both sides of the backbone, and discard it. Use the heel of your hand to press down on the breastbone to open it up.

Pierce the chicken a few times with a sharp knife, especially over the legs and breast, to help it cook evenly.

Put the chillies (remove the stems first), tomatoes, garlic, lemon juice, vinegar, parsley, paprika, oregano, sugar and salt into a blender and blitz until smooth.

Spread the marinade all over the chicken, then cover and leave to marinate in the fridge for an hour.

Preheat the oven to 210°C fan/450°F/gas mark 8.

Uncover the chicken, place it in a roasting tray, breast side up, and cook for 50–60 minutes, or until the juices run clear.

Once cooked, place the chicken under a high grill for a few minutes to char the skin. Remove from the grill, cover with foil and leave to rest for 10 minutes.

NOTES

The choice of chillies will determine how hot this is – pick ones to your liking.

If freezing, do it before cooking.

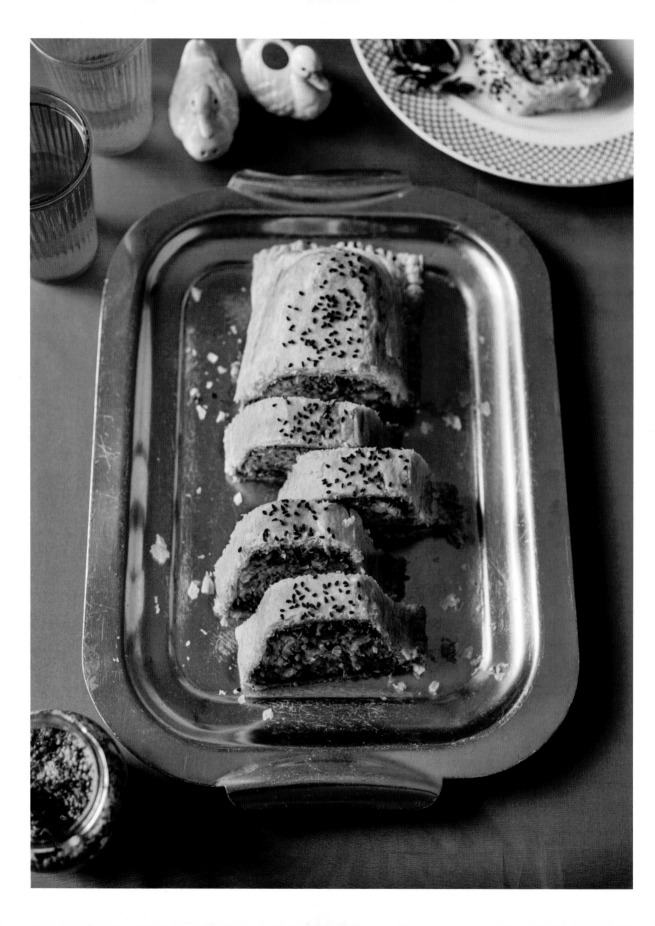

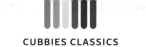
NOT-QUITE-BEEF WELLINGTON

Beef Wellington is quite possibly one of our favourite things to order when we're eating out, and we oh-so-wanted to do it for this book. However, it's been done, and we wanted a decent vegetarian recipe as a replacement. It took some faffing and farting about, but we got there in the end and are frankly delighted with the results.

SERVES: 6
PREP: 30 minutes
COOK: 1 hour 20 minutes
CALORIES: 462

For the duxelles

500g (1lb 2oz) mushrooms, finely chopped
1 onion, finely chopped
1 clove of garlic, crushed or grated
1 teaspoon dried rosemary

For the Wellington

1 onion, finely chopped
1 celery stalk, chopped
300g (10½oz) button mushrooms, finely chopped
2 cloves of garlic, crushed or grated
2 × 400g (14oz) tins of chickpeas, drained and rinsed
100g (3½oz) panko breadcrumbs
45g (1½oz) porridge oats
1 teaspoon salt
1 teaspoon black pepper
1 teaspoon dried mixed herbs
1 teaspoon dried rosemary
3 tablespoons soy sauce
3 tablespoons tomato sauce
½ teaspoon dried chilli flakes
1 × 375g (13oz) sheet of light puff pastry
2 tablespoons milk
1 teaspoon black onion seeds

Spray a large frying pan with a little oil and place over a medium heat. Add the duxelles ingredients and gently cook until all the liquid has evaporated, about 20–30 minutes, stirring frequently. Remove from the heat and set aside.

Preheat the oven to 180°C fan/400°F/gas mark 6 and line a baking tray with greaseproof paper.

Spray another frying pan with a little oil and place over a medium-high heat. Add the onion, celery, button mushrooms and garlic and cook for about 5 minutes, then set aside.

Tip the drained chickpeas into a food processor and pulse until you have a chunky texture (or alternatively mash with a fork). Transfer to a bowl.

Add the panko breadcrumbs, porridge oats, salt, pepper, mixed herbs, rosemary, soy sauce, tomato sauce and chilli flakes and mix well until combined.

Tip out the chickpea mix on to a piece of clingfilm and form into a meatloaf shape, then wrap and place in the fridge for 30 minutes to firm up.

Meanwhile, roll out the sheet of puff pastry so that it fits a 24cm × 18cm (9½ inch × 7 inch) baking tray, and spread with a layer of the (cooled) duxelles mix.

Remove the chickpea loaf from the fridge, gently unwrap, and place in the middle of the sheet. Spread the rest of the duxelles mix over the log as best you can, then gently bring the pastry up over the sides, and crimp together.

Brush the pastry with a little milk and sprinkle over the onion seeds.

Bake in the oven for 45 minutes. Then slice and serve!

NOTE

We appreciate this is a bit of a clart on for a TCC recipe, but we promise it's worth it!

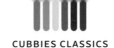

BREAKFAST BOMB

Yep, a breakfast bomb in a book about easy evening meals – I bet it's all you can do not to get on your soapbox and fire off an angry letter at us. We understand: it's the lies you can't handle. But here's the thing: James came up with it when he was hungover and hanging out of his a*se, which always means he doesn't get out of bed until the early evening anyway, so suck it. We're calling it a breakfast bomb because it uses all the ingredients you would expect in a fry-up made into this absolute beast. It's excellent for using up a stray egg here, a packet of sausages there.

You can swap most of the ingredients out and substitute more of the others if there's any you don't fancy. For example, Paul doesn't like black pudding, so I leave it out. Paul, that is, not the black pudding. To really twist the knife, I make him peer in through the cat-flap while I eat his portion and cackle maniacally. It's a hard life.

Oh, and I'm not going to fib here: this looks bloody terrible. But just trust me. Pure stodge.

SERVES: 4
PREP: 10 minutes
COOK: 50 minutes
CALORIES: 371

1 × 440g (14oz) tin of baked beans
1 small tin of mushrooms, drained and chopped finely
½ × 400g (14oz) tin of chopped tomatoes
4 low-fat Cumberland sausages
2 thick slices of black pudding
2 large eggs
8 rashers of back bacon (unsmoked or smoked, your choice, but you want rashers with plenty of meat on them)

Preheat the oven to an entirely modest 170°C fan/375°F/gas mark 5. Spray the inside of a hemisphere cake pan (or see notes) with some olive oil, then brush it around with a pastry brush – every nook and cranny. Set it to one side.

Get the beans, mushrooms and tomatoes into a pan spit-spot and have them simmer away on the hob until the sauce is reduced and claggy, like proper school-dinner beans.

Cook your sausages in a frying pan, and when they're almost done, pop the black pudding into the same pan and cook until crispy.

Take your beans off the hob and crack 2 eggs into them, stirring all the while until all is mixed in.

Chop your sausages and one of the slices of black pudding into little chunks and stir into the beans.

Take your bacon and line the inside of your cake pan (imagine you're creating half a football – you want no cracks if you can help it), with enough hanging over to put over the top.

Place the second disc of black pudding at the bottom of the tin.

Fill with the bean and tomato filling and pack it down, then fold the bacon over the top and press down.

Wrap the whole thing in foil and cook in the oven for about 15 minutes.

Check the bacon is cooked and if it is, tip the breakfast bomb out on to a plate, let it cool, then slice and serve.

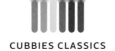
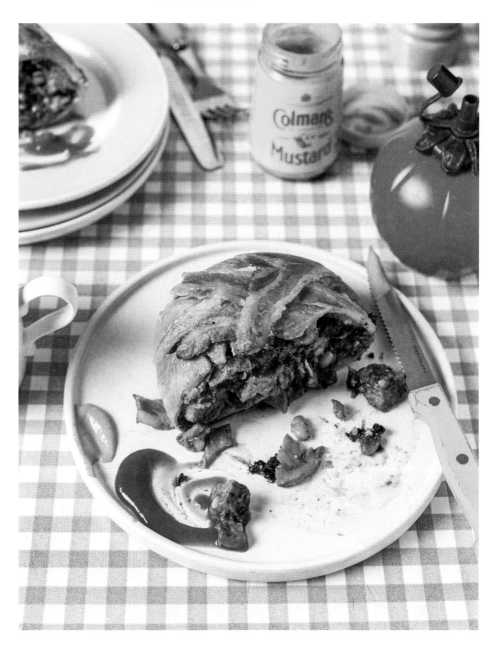

NOTES

A hemisphere cake pan can be found in most supermarkets and baking stores, but if you don't have one, fret not – you can use a normal Pyrex casserole dish and muddle through. The pan we use is 16cm across and comes from Lakeland.

You might want to buy a second pack of bacon in case you need a couple of rashers extra to wrap this all up – and think, you can have yourself a bacon sandwich while this cooks to really give the ambulance crew something to laugh about while they pop you on the stretcher.

If you want a cheaper option, you could use slices of ham for the outside, but layer it a few times, otherwise it'll burn.

Leftover filling can be frozen for another time – and you can make smaller versions by using a muffin tin, lining the gaps with ham and making parcels.

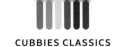
CHICKEN LASAGNE

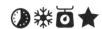

This is a long recipe, so let's keep the intro as short as we can, shall we? It's a classic from the blog that people tend to avoid because it seems a little out there, but we implore you to give it a go: it's utterly divine.

Speaking of the blog, it is utterly crazy to think that nine years ago (at the time of writing) we thought it would be a good idea to waffle on about our slimming class and expect people to read. We never forget that, and those who have been with us from the beginning. A tiny plea though: if you're familiar with us through the books alone, take a look at twochubbycubs.com – there's over 750 more recipes on there now, and nine years' worth of writing. Fill your boots! To the lasagne then – enjoy!

SERVES: 4
PREP: 10 minutes
COOK: 1 hour 20 minutes
CALORIES: 500

2 leeks, finely sliced
450g (1lb) chicken mince
4 cloves of garlic, crushed
    or grated
1 teaspoon dried oregano
1 teaspoon dried sage
1 × 400g (14oz) tin of chopped
    tomatoes
3 tablespoons passata
2 tablespoons tomato purée
200g (7oz) frozen peas
1 tablespoon Worcestershire
    sauce
200g (7oz) ricotta
15g (½oz) Parmesan cheese,
    grated
8–12 lasagne sheets
12 cherry tomatoes
55g (2oz) reduced-fat mozzarella
salt and black pepper

Preheat the oven to 180°C fan/400°F/gas mark 6.

Place a large frying pan over a medium-low heat and spray with a little oil. Add the leeks and cook until softened, about 8–10 minutes.

Increase the heat to medium, add the chicken mince and garlic, and cook until the meat is no longer pink, stirring frequently.

Add the oregano, sage, chopped tomatoes, passata and tomato purée, along with 4 tablespoons of water. Add the frozen peas and Worcestershire sauce and season with salt and pepper. Bring to the boil, then simmer for 10–15 minutes.

Meanwhile, put the ricotta and Parmesan into a small saucepan and warm over a low heat until the ricotta softens.

Spoon one third of the chicken mix into the bottom of an ovenproof dish, followed by a third of the cheesy sauce and a layer of lasagne sheets. Repeat with two more layers.

Arrange the cherry tomatoes in a fancy manner on top, and place torn-up chunks of mozzarella in between.

Bake in the oven for 35 minutes.

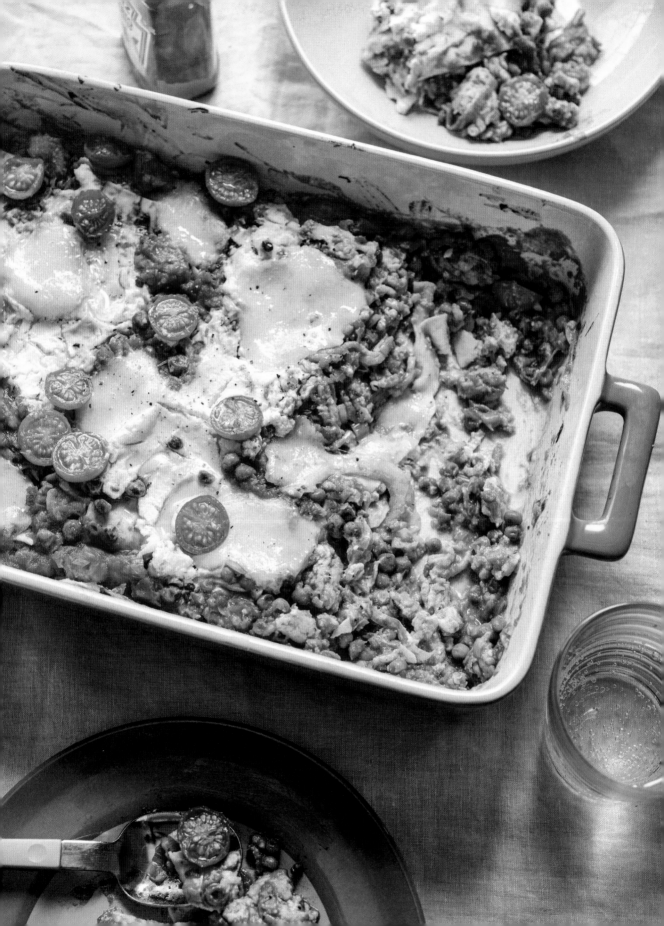

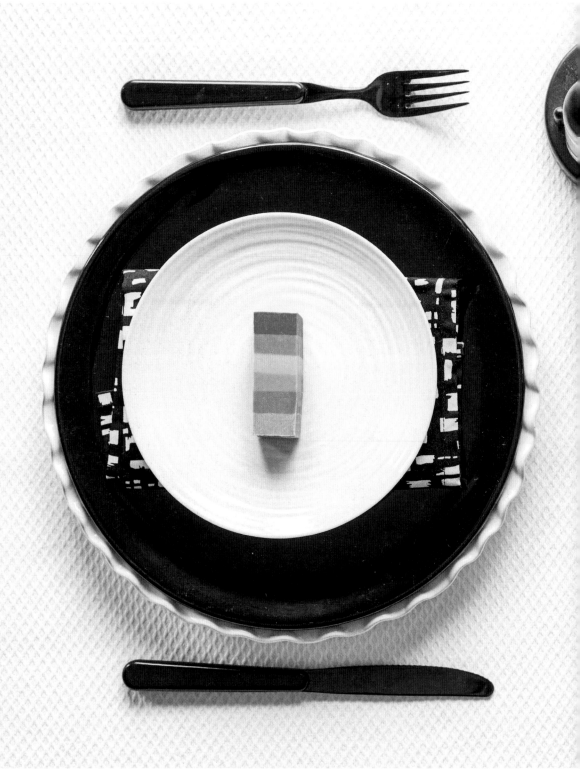

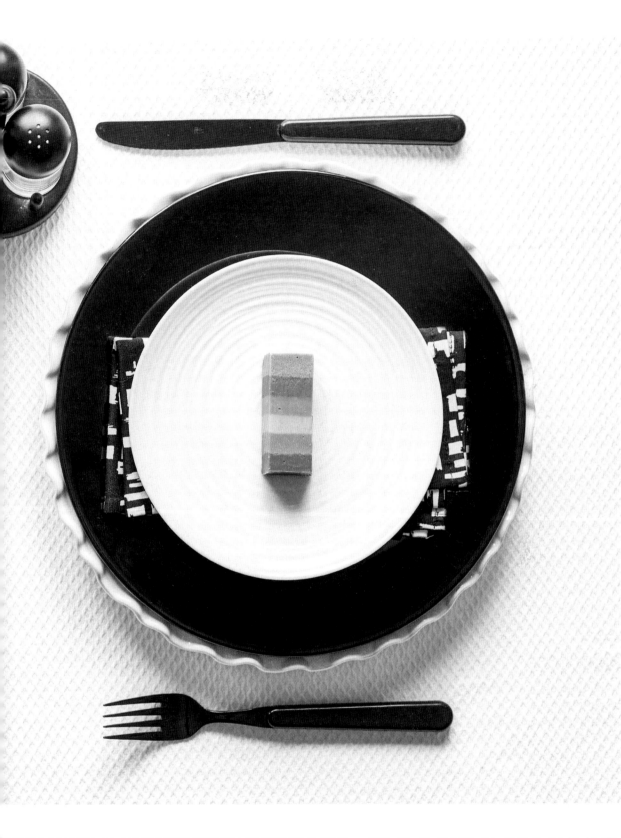

FAKEAWAYS

FAMOUS SWEDISH SHOP MEATBALLS & GRAVY

But which famous shop could we possibly mean? That's right! We've perfectly replicated the H&M meatballs experience! Well no, of course not, we're speaking of the wonderful blue warehouse of budget furniture, tasteful decoration and endless acrimony. I simply refuse to visit with Paul because we both know how it will end – a huge argument, a terse drive home and one of us moving out for a couple of days because we disagreed on what colour draining-rack to buy. We once made the error of purchasing our kitchen through their excellent design service. I had to confess to three affairs to calm the situation down afterwards.

No couple, friendship or acquaintanceship has ever survived more than twenty minutes in there, and to claim otherwise is a fib. I'm starting to suspect that they pump testosterone through the air-vents (TESTOSTERON is probably the name of a side table you can buy).

However, there is one light at the end of the tunnel and it's the meatballs. In much the same style as a Costco hotdog, any trip has to include a plate of these, dolloped with lingonberry jam. We can't pretend these are identical, but they're so, so close.

SERVES: 4
PREP: 15 minutes
COOK: 20 minutes
CALORIES: 208

500g (1lb 2oz) turkey mince
1 teaspoon fresh rosemary leaves
1 teaspoon fresh oregano leaves
1 teaspoon paprika
1 clove of garlic, crushed or grated
salt and black pepper
1 tablespoon fresh parsley, chopped
½ teaspoon nutmeg
2 tablespoons low-fat soft cheese
2 beef stock cubes, dissolved in 450ml (16fl oz) boiling water
1 teaspoon mustard powder
1 tablespoon Worcestershire sauce
1 tablespoon cornflour
gherkins, to serve (optional)

In a bowl mix together the mince, rosemary, oregano, paprika, garlic, salt, pepper, half the parsley and half the nutmeg, and roll into about 30 meatballs.

Spray a large frying pan with a little oil and place on a medium-high heat. Add the meatballs and cook until browned and no pink meat remains, then transfer to a plate and keep warm.

Add the soft cheese and 2 tablespoons of beef stock to the pan and mix well until the cheese has softened and melted.

Add the mustard powder, Worcestershire sauce, cornflour and the rest of the nutmeg, and mix well until you have a smooth, thick paste.

Add the rest of the stock and cook over a low heat, stirring continuously until it thickens.

Serve the meatballs, pour over the gravy and scatter the remaining parsley over the top.

NOTES

Have this with whatever you like, but really, it has to be chips, doesn't it? Mash is lovely too.

If you don't have fresh oregano and rosemary, don't sweat it – ¼ teaspoon of each dried will work just as well.

If you're freezing, just freeze the meatballs and make the gravy fresh.

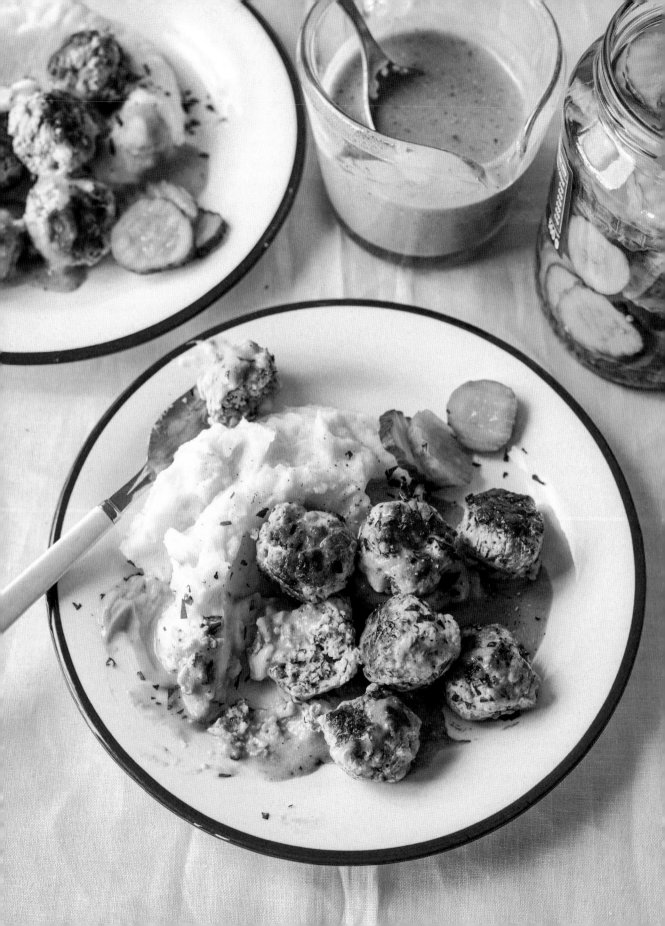

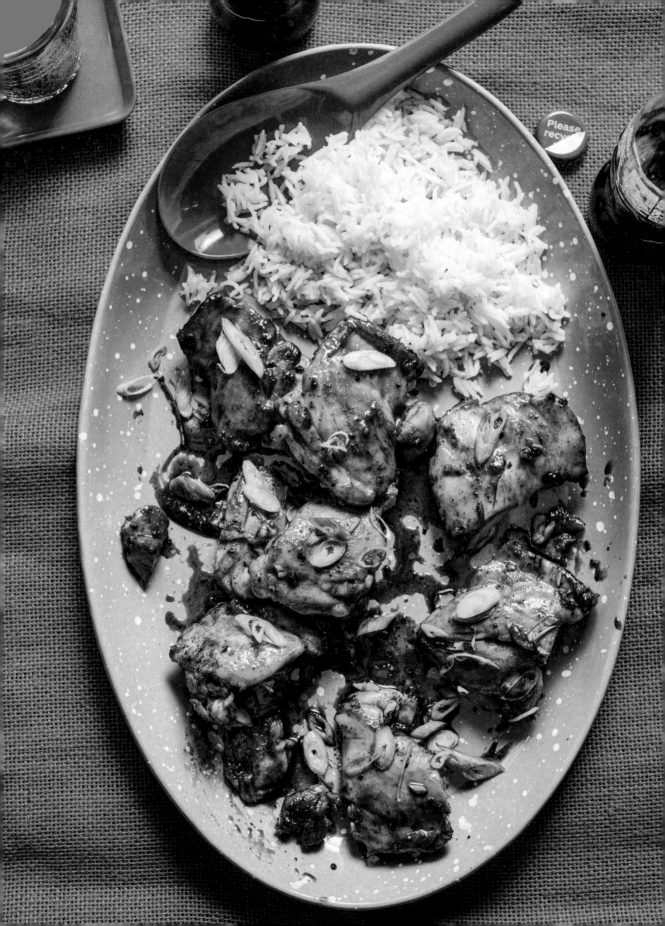

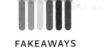
SWEET & SOUR COLA CHICKEN

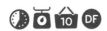

Although chicken cooked in cola has been doing the rounds on the Internet ever since the dancing hamster was a thing and I was optimistically describing myself as 'defined' on my dating profiles, we have never committed our own version to print. For this recipe we have made it more of a sweet and sour sauce and we will not apologise for this: it's a sticky, saucy delight.

Although Paul cautions this in the notes, I am going to put it right here at the top too: please do not use diet cola. Just don't. The sugar is a key part of this, and given it still comes in under 500 calories you have no excuse not to treat yourself. We have seen some hot-takes using tropical pop too – readers, you mustn't. We are normally all for encouraging experimentation – your husband says hi and he won't be home tonight – but no. Not like this.

SERVES: 4
PREP: 5 minutes
COOK: 30 minutes
MARINATING: 1 hour
CALORIES: 301

600g (1lb 5oz) skinless, boneless
   chicken thighs
2 tablespoons white wine
2cm (¾ inch) piece of root ginger,
   thinly sliced
3 cloves of garlic, thinly sliced
1 teaspoon light soy sauce
1 teaspoon dark soy sauce
1 teaspoon salt
500ml (18fl oz) cola
2 spring onions, finely sliced

Place everything but the spring onions in a bowl, cover with cling film (or a sealable bag), and leave to marinate for an hour.

Remove the chicken, shake off any excess and set aside.

Pour the marinade into a saucepan and bring to the boil over a medium-high heat. Reduce the heat to a simmer and cook until there's about 125ml (4fl oz) left (about half a mugful), then set aside.

Meanwhile, spray a large frying pan with a little oil and place over a medium-high heat. Open out the chicken thighs and put them into the pan, then cook for 10–15 minutes, until no pink meat remains.

Increase the heat to high, then pour in the reduced marinade and stir until the chicken is well coated.

Serve the chicken on a plate, pour over the remaining marinade, and sprinkle over the spring onions.

NOTES

Don't be tempted to use diet cola for this – it won't work as well.

You can use chicken breasts if you prefer, but really, thighs are best.

This is great with rice, chips, or whatever you fancy!

PAD KRAPOW

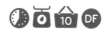

We did a version of pad krapow so many moons ago on the blog and then, like a lot of our early recipes, completely forgot about it. Looking back, we served this on glass noodles which, although tasty, don't exactly look great – so this is a new, improved version that we hope will tickle your pickle. If not, there's an absolutely wonderful Thai restaurant up here in Newcastle and we're sure they'll knock you out a charming version should you ask. If you want the name, send us a message – I'm not putting the name here because we don't want it overrun: it's the perfect place to end up after the cinema and you can always get a seat at the moment. So, we love you, but stay away.

Thai food is just the thing to take the edge off going to the cinema, though, given that's become an exercise in frustration and anger. No room for a rant here, but just know this: if you're the sort of person who gets their phone out at *any* point past the trailers, I'll take great delight in sucking the chocolate off a Malteser and throwing the soggy honeycomb into your hair.

SERVES: 4
PREP: 35 minutes
COOK: 20 minutes
CALORIES: 494

6 tablespoons oyster sauce
600g (1lb 5oz) skinless, boneless
    chicken thighs, diced
225g (8oz) jasmine rice
4 cloves of garlic, crushed
    or grated
4 red chillies, finely chopped
2 teaspoons dark soy sauce
2 teaspoons light soy sauce
1 teaspoon sugar
30g (1oz) Thai basil
4 eggs

Spread the oyster sauce over the chicken thighs and leave to marinate for 30 minutes.

Bring a large pan of water to the boil and add the rice. Put a lid on the pan, reduce the heat to low, cook for 10 minutes, then drain and return the rice to the pan to steam.

Meanwhile, spray a large frying pan with a little oil and place over a high heat. Add the chicken and cook for 5–6 minutes.

Add the garlic and chillies and cook for another minute. Add the soy sauces and sugar and stir well. Reduce the heat to medium, add the basil leaves and cook until wilted.

Spoon the chicken over the rice and place the pan back over the heat.

Crack in the eggs and cook for 2 minutes, then serve on top of the chicken and rice.

NOTES

Can't find Thai basil? Normal basil will be OK to use instead.

Chicken breast is fine to use if you prefer.

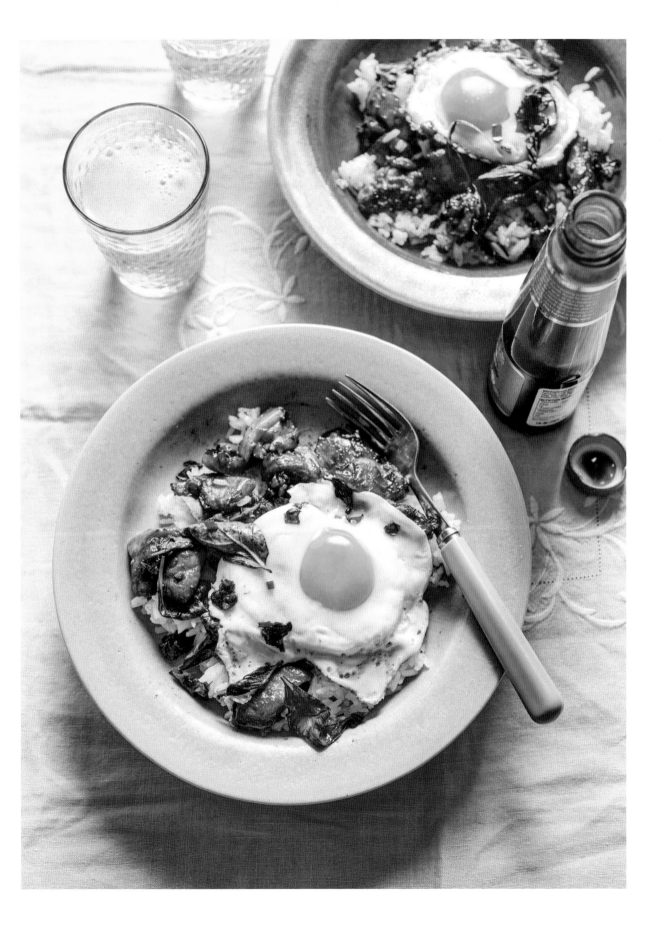

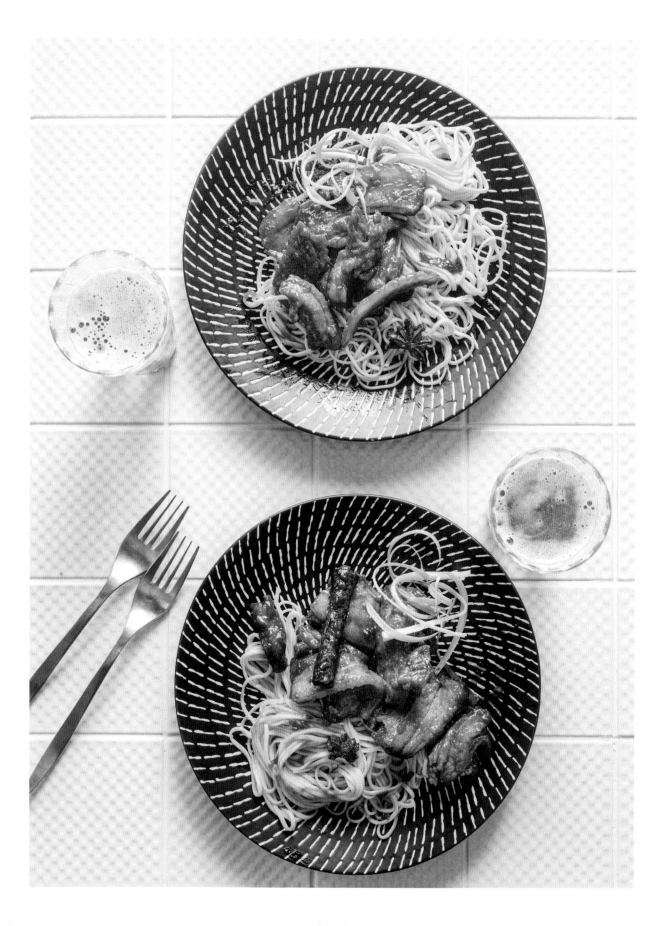

JAMES'S STICKY PORK BELLY

You might be thinking that those simpering balls of giggles at twochubbycubs have only put this sticky pork belly recipe in so they can include a title that sounds like a filthy joke – and you would be right. Given my belly looks like a glazed doughnut that has rolled across the floor of a barbershop at the best of times, it seemed only fitting.

But, smutty title aside, this is actually one of those recipes which a lot of people will instinctively avoid if they're on a diet. Pork belly does have a lot of fat, but see, it's the fat that makes this delicious. We've always been of the mind that a little of what you fancy does you good, and never more so than when it comes to cooking. Fat and sugar must never be the enemy of the dieter: when used correctly they add flavour and depth to a dish. Various slimming clubs and diet plans will tell you otherwise, but we say they can bore off. When have we ever steered you wrong?

SERVES: 4
PREP: 10 minutes
COOK: 1 hour 45 minutes
CALORIES: 365

500g (1lb 2oz) pork belly
2 tablespoons + 2 teaspoons rice
    wine vinegar
1 tablespoon + 1 teaspoon dark
    soy sauce
1 shallot, finely diced
2 tablespoons light soy sauce
1 tablespoon honey
1 cinnamon stick
2 star anise
3 spring onions, sliced

Slice the pork belly into small strips. Place in a sandwich bag with 2 teaspoons of rice wine vinegar and 1 teaspoon of dark soy sauce, and leave to marinate for an hour.

Place a frying pan or a wok over a medium heat and spray with a little oil. Add the shallot and fry for 3–4 minutes, until lightly browned.

Add the pork belly strips and cook for 5 minutes, until they too are starting to brown, then add the rest of the rice wine vinegar and dark soy sauce, the light soy sauce, honey, cinnamon stick and star anise and mix well.

Add 200ml (7fl oz) of water, stir and bring to the boil, then reduce the heat to low and cover with a lid. Leave to simmer for 1 hour, then remove from the heat.

Serve the pork over rice or noodles, sprinkled with the sliced spring onions.

NACHO NORMAL PEPPER DISH

You have no idea how long I agonised trying to make a nacho/macho man pun work in that title, but I just couldn't do it. To be fair, the title is irrelevant when compared to just how good this recipe is: it takes one of my most favourite foods (nachos) and turns it into a full dish of its own. Which is lucky because, quite frankly, the United Kingdom can simply not do nachos justice. I've railed against this injustice a few times but I'm now throwing it open to our readers – if you can recommend somewhere in the UK whose nachos dish is more than a packet of Doritos that someone waved a Babybel at and then microwaved, get in touch with us and we'll go visit. But if you let me down, well …

SERVES: 4
PREP: 15 minutes
COOK: 1 hour
CALORIES: 491

1 pouch of microwave wholegrain rice
3 peppers (any colour)
200g (7oz) lean beef mince
200g (7oz) pork mince
2 teaspoons hot chilli powder
½ teaspoon ground cumin
½ teaspoon paprika
¼ teaspoon dried chilli flakes
1 tablespoon onion granules
1 × 300g (10½oz) jar of salsa
225ml (7½fl oz) passata

Toppings

50g (1¾oz) tortilla crisps, crushed
¼ iceberg lettuce, sliced
a handful of black olives, sliced
8 cherry tomatoes, quartered
4 tablespoons reduced-fat crème fraîche
4 tablespoons sliced jalapeños, drained
4 tablespoons (60g/ 2¼oz) reduced-fat Cheddar cheese, grated
1 bunch of fresh coriander, roughly chopped

Preheat the oven to 180°C fan/400°F/gas mark 6.

Heat the microwave rice according to the instructions, then tip into a large bowl and leave to cool for a few minutes.

Slice each pepper in half and remove the core and seeds, then place in an ovenproof dish (cut side up).

Add the mince, chilli powder, cumin, paprika, chilli flakes, onion granules and half the salsa to the rice and mix well.

Divide the mixture into 6 and stuff into the pepper halves.

In another bowl, mix together the passata and the remaining salsa and spoon over the peppers. Pour 100ml (3½fl oz) of water into the bottom of the dish (careful not to wash away any of the tomato mix) and cover with foil or a lid.

Bake in the oven for 1 hour, then remove from the oven and leave to rest for 10 minutes.

Divide the toppings between the peppers, and serve.

NOTE

Not a fan of microwave rice? Any cooked rice will be fine – we just like to cut corners!

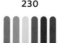

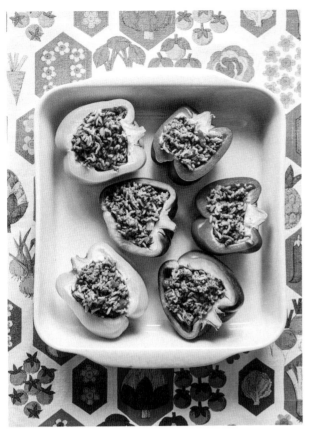

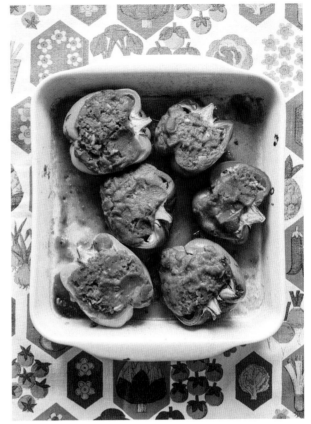

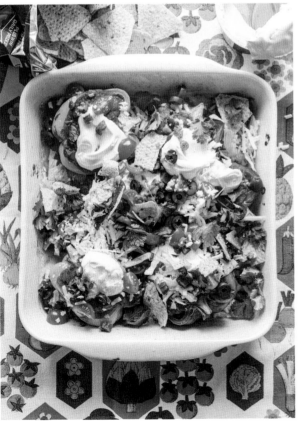

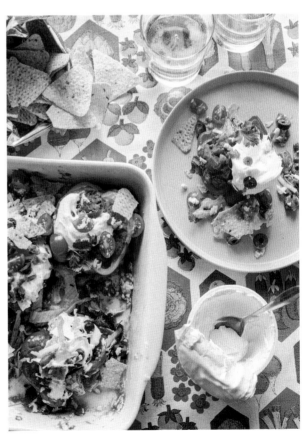

PEKING SHREDDED PORK

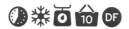

We're making absolutely no claim as to the authenticity of this dish – and to be fair, we never do for any of our dishes, as we're very aware that we are two uncultured swines from the land of the Stottie – but we can promise you it is absolutely, utterly magnificent.

Peking anything always reminds me of my mate Tim, who I used to visit in London for weeks at a time when I was a teenager. I led a very Tracy Barlow life at home in rural Northumberland, in that my parents always just assumed I was upstairs listening to my tapes, and so going to the capital was therefore always terrifically exciting.

Tim is a walking encyclopedia when it comes to Asian cuisine and we ate in some lovely places as a result, though perhaps my most prevailing memory of him was the time we went to Nancy Lam's Enak Enak restaurant for dinner. Nancy herself was hosting, and the moment we squeezed into her bustling restaurant, she dashed over and sat us right by the front door. When we asked why, she looked us up and down appraisingly and declared we needed the cool air as we were so very, *very* fat.

To be fair to her honesty, neither of us had missed many meals, but even so.

SERVES: 4
PREP: 30 minutes
COOK: 15 minutes
CALORIES: 207

500g (1lb 2oz) pork tenderloin
4 spring onions, sliced

For the marinade
4 tablespoons rice wine
2 tablespoons soy sauce
1 teaspoon bicarbonate of soda
    (mixed with 2 tablespoons
    water)
1 teaspoon cornflour

For the sauce
3 tablespoons hoisin sauce
4 teaspoons sugar
1 teaspoon cornflour (mixed with
    2 tablespoons water)

Whisk together the marinade ingredients in a large bowl.

Slice the tenderloin into thin strips and add to the marinade, tossing to coat, then cover with clingfilm and leave for 15–20 minutes.

Meanwhile, whisk together all the sauce ingredients and set aside.

Spray a large wok or frying pan with a little oil and place over a medium-high heat. Add the pork and any remaining marinade and cook until no pink meat remains. Scoop the pork from the pan and keep warm.

Pour the sauce ingredients into the pan, reduce the heat to medium and simmer until thickened.

Put the pork back into the pan and toss to coat with the sauce.

Serve the pork sprinkled with the sliced spring onions.

NOTES

This is also great made with beef, or even chicken!

If freezing, do it once the pork is cooked and before you make the sauce.

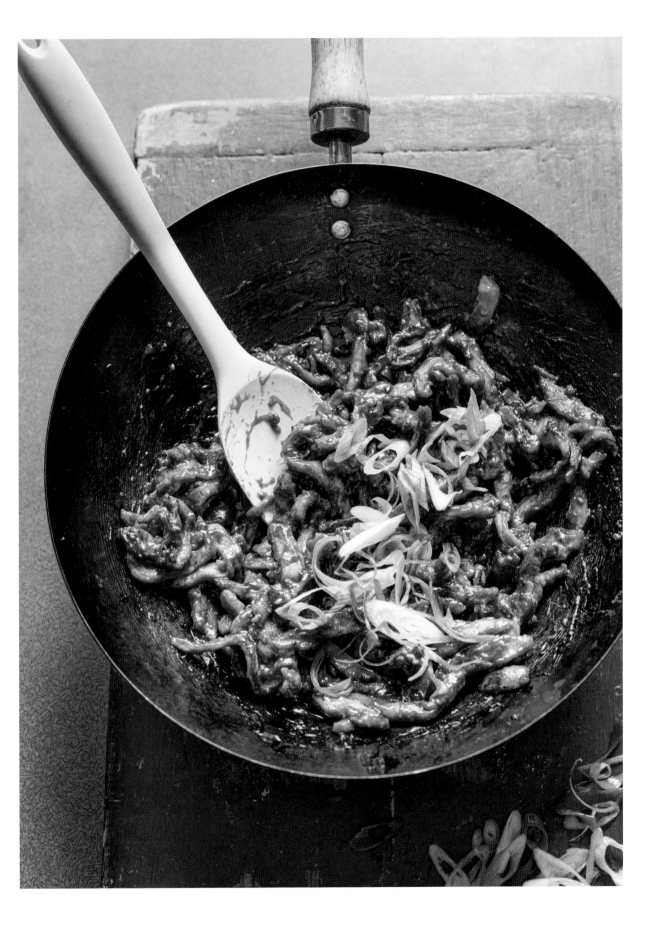

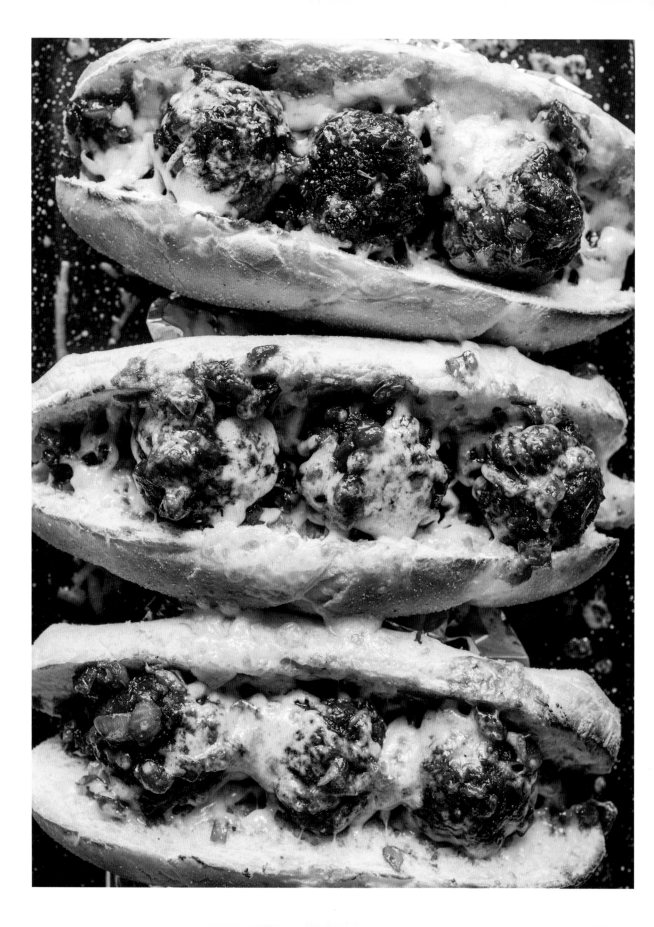

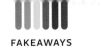
MEATBALL SUB

There's a chain of sandwich shops which we can't possibly name but who do the most amazing meatball subs – a giant sandwich where you have to dislocate your jaw to get it all in. Well, I don't, but I've had several years of stretching my mouth open to accommodate something meaty. Anyway, we've replicated the experience here the best we can, but of course, if you want the real thing, you'll need to stand in front of your kitchen counter looking dazed and confused while someone fresh into puberty mumbles your salad choices back at you.

Way back when, in the first flush of my teenage years, I was merrily drunk on too many Incredible Hulks (lager and blue WKD) and when it came to my drunken takeaway order, could I buggery remember the word teriyaki. Still, I'm sure the sight of some twenty-stone chancer yelling 'CHICKEN TICKY-LICKY PLEASE' and then falling over must have brought joy to their lives.

SERVES: 4
PREP: 15 minutes
COOK: 1 hour 15 minutes
CALORIES: 498

250g (9oz) lean beef mince
250g (9oz) pork mince
25g (1oz) panko breadcrumbs
1 egg
1 onion, diced
300ml (10fl oz) ale
50g (1¾oz) brown sugar
1 teaspoon salt
1 teaspoon dried thyme
1 teaspoon paprika
1 teaspoon mustard powder
1 teaspoon garlic granules
¼ teaspoon black pepper
4 submarine buns
60g (2¼oz) Cheddar cheese, grated

In a bowl, mix together the beef and pork mince along with the panko breadcrumbs and the egg. Roll the mixture into 12 balls.

Spray a large casserole dish with a little oil and place over a medium-high heat. Add the meatballs and cook until browned all over.

Meanwhile, whisk together the onion, ale, sugar, salt, thyme, paprika, mustard powder, garlic granules and pepper. Reduce the heat under the casserole to low, then pour the mix into the pan of meatballs. Stir gently, then cover with a lid and simmer for 1 hour, stirring occasionally.

When the meatballs are cooked, remove from the heat and preheat the grill to medium-high.

Slice the buns horizontally and add 3 meatballs to each one, then sprinkle over the cheese and place on a grill pan (try to lay the subs on their 'spine' if you can).

Grill for 4–5 minutes, until the cheese is melted and golden.

Serve!

NOTES

If you can't find submarine rolls, hot dog rolls will do, or any other kind – it doesn't really matter.

Only the meatballs are suitable for freezing.

BUTTER PANEER

Paneer is one of those ingredients that seem to mystify people: like the orzo from previous books, almost. It's essentially just cottage cheese, but is usually sold as one solid block, and although it doesn't taste of anything on its own (taking the title as the only cheese we can safely leave in the fridge without finding giant tooth-bites in it from Paul's midnight snacking), it carries flavour ever so well. Of course, if you're not a fan of paneer you can always swap it out for chicken breast, but we encourage you to give it a go if you're sitting on the fence.

I can see Paul has noted this below, but it bears repeating: please do not use fat-free yoghurt. For those few calories you save you run the risk of ruining the dish with a split yoghurt, and while split yoghurt doesn't impair the flavour of the dish, it does make it look like something the dog left on the carpet.

SERVES: 4
PREP: 10 minutes
COOK: 25 minutes
CALORIES: 499

4 cloves of garlic, crushed
  or grated
170g (6oz) Greek yoghurt
1 teaspoon ground turmeric
2 teaspoons garam masala
1 teaspoon ground coriander
½ teaspoon paprika
2½cm (1 inch) piece of root
  ginger, grated
juice of ½ lemon
400g (14oz) paneer, cut into
  2cm cubes
1½ tablespoons butter
1 teaspoon salt
400ml (14fl oz) passata
115g (4oz) low-fat soft cheese
1 bunch of fresh coriander,
  chopped

In a bowl, mix together the garlic, yoghurt, turmeric, garam masala, ground coriander, paprika, ginger and lemon juice.

Add the paneer to the bowl and gently stir until well combined.

Spray a large frying pan with a little oil and place over a medium heat. Add the butter and stir until melted.

Add the paneer to the pan with all the marinade and cook for 4–5 minutes.

Add the salt, passata and soft cheese to the pan, stir, then bring to a simmer for 20 minutes.

Serve with rice and sprinkle with the chopped coriander.

NOTES

Don't use fat-free yoghurt for this. Only the good stuff will do.

Quorn, tofu and chicken all work just as well in this, but we really love paneer.

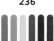

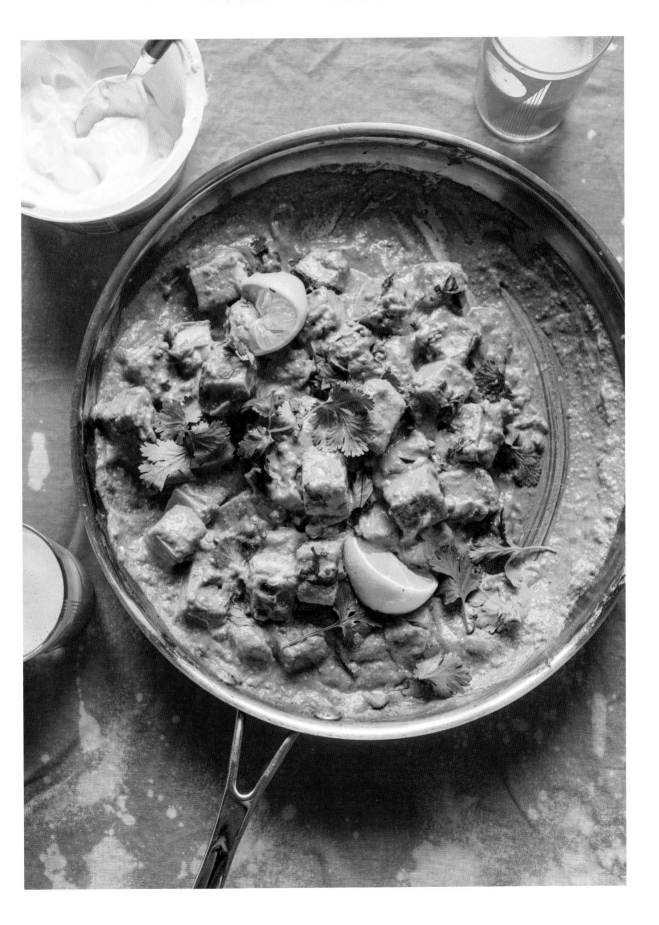

CUB-FIL-A CRISPY CHICKEN SANDWICH

This is a little holdover from our minces around America, where good fried chicken can be found everywhere you look. You can't beat a good crunchy chicken sandwich, and that's a fact. Paul suggests chicken breasts to keep things simple, but I shall interject with the plea to get yourself some boneless thighs and savour the flavour! TESTIFY!

I apologise, I got carried away there.

Of course, as delicious as this sandwich is, it pales in comparison to the best food to ever come out of America: blue raspberry Jolly Ranchers. If you think I'm naming them in an utterly shameless bid to get a free truckload of them sent to my house, well, you're absolutely bloody right.

Sandwich, anyone?

SERVES: 4
PREP: 10 minutes
COOK: 25 minutes
CALORIES: 445

60g (2¼oz) panko breadcrumbs
¼ teaspoon salt
¼ teaspoon black pepper
1 teaspoon dried basil
4 skinless, boneless chicken breasts
1 egg, beaten
2 tablespoons reduced-fat mayonnaise
5 tablespoons reduced-fat sour cream
1 teaspoon sriracha
½ teaspoon paprika
4 buns
8 sliced gherkins

Preheat the oven to 220°C fan/475°F/gas mark 9 and line a baking sheet with greaseproof paper.

Mix the panko breadcrumbs with the salt, pepper and dried basil. Dip the chicken into the beaten egg, then dredge through the panko breadcrumbs until well coated and place on the baking sheet.

Bake in the oven for 25 minutes.

Meanwhile, mix together the mayonnaise, sour cream, sriracha and paprika and set aside.

Slice the buns in half, spray with a little oil, and toast.

Spread a little sauce on to the bottom half of each bun and top with a chicken breast, some gherkins and a little more sauce, followed by the top half of each bun.

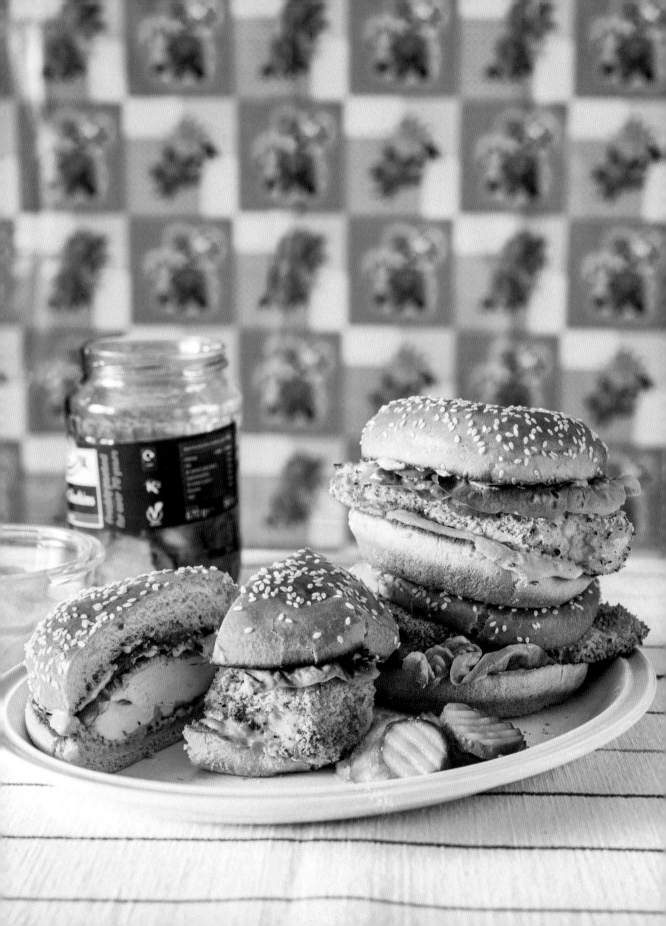

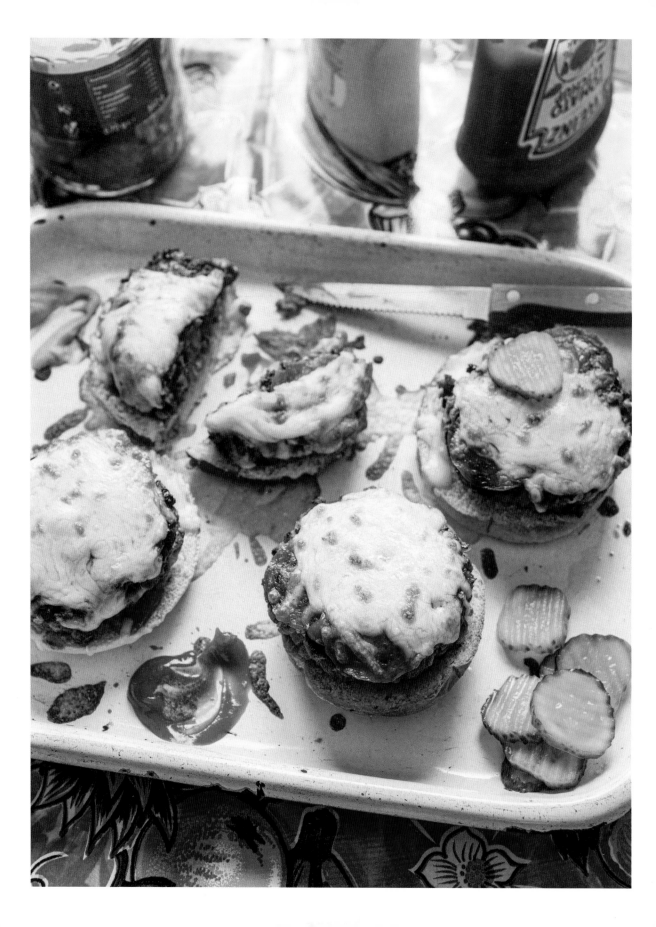

BURGER PIZZAS

This burger pizza is a slightly lighter take on our 'Dirty Threesome' burger from the blog (which we encourage you to quickly Google, because it is tremendous) and combines all the good bits of a pizza with the meaty goodness of a burger. The 'Dirty Threesome' combined a burger, chips, chilli and pizza bits into one almighty stack of calories, and although this is a slightly more muted affair, it's still going to trouble your jaw in all the best ways.

Oh, and just so you know, our burger position still hasn't changed over the last few years: if you can't fit it comfortably in your mouth without having to take it apart, then it's not a burger. It's an endurance test, albeit a delicious one.

MAKES: 4
PREP: 10 minutes
COOK: 18 minutes
CALORIES: 415

2 burger buns
1 onion, finely chopped
2 cloves of garlic, crushed
　or grated
400g (14oz) lean minced beef
½ teaspoon dried oregano
3 tablespoons tomato purée,
　mixed with 4 tablespoons
　water
8 pepperoni slices
150g (5½oz) grated mozzarella
　cheese
gherkins, to serve (optional)

Slice the buns in half, then toast them in a toaster and set aside.

Spray a large frying pan with a little oil. Add the onion and garlic and cook for 4–5 minutes, until softened and turning golden.

Put the mince into a large bowl, add the fried onions and the oregano, and mix well to combine.

Divide the mixture into 4 balls and flatten into burgers. Put the burgers back into the pan and cook for 6–7 minutes, turning them every minute.

Meanwhile, put the bun halves on a baking sheet, cut side up, and preheat the grill to high.

Place the burgers on top of the buns and top each one with the tomato sauce, 2 slices of pepperoni and a sprinkling of mozzarella.

Place under the hot grill and cook for 3–4 minutes, until the cheese has melted and is bubbling.

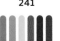

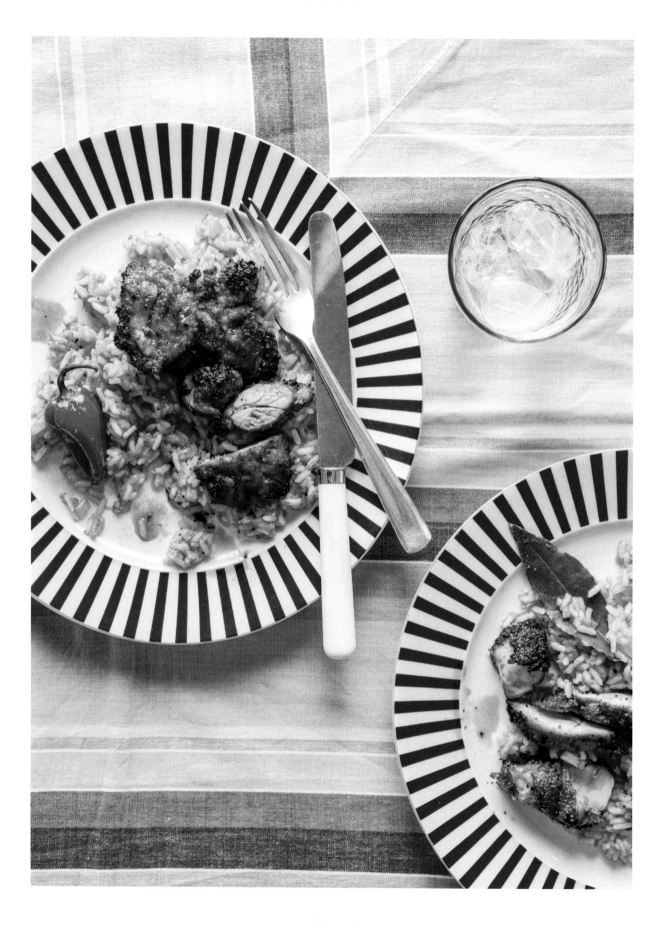

JOLLOF RICE

This recipe was recommended to us as one to try by one of Paul's work colleagues. We didn't take much persuasion, but then neither of us ever do. Jollof rice is a Nigerian recipe that combines spice, rice and chicken into a delicious, slightly ring-troubling one-pan dish.

All for one-pan dishes in this household, not least because the loading of the dishwasher is always an exercise in me jamming everything in like a glitched game of Tetris, and Paul coming in later and icily informing me that nothing has been cleaned because the spinny-doohickey thing couldn't turn. How we laugh at my incompetence, but I'll admit something here: I'm just playing the long game. I can't abide loading the dishwasher and I'm hoping that if I do it badly enough times, Paul will give in and do it himself.

Of course, if he's doing his job of proofreading these intros, then my plan falls apart. But know this, reader, if you're reading this, then that means he didn't and my evil plan continues. Care to join me for a cackle?

SERVES: 4
PREP: 10 minutes
COOK: 1 hour 10 minutes
CALORIES: 483

6 skinless, boneless chicken
    thighs
1 tablespoon paprika
2 teaspoons onion granules
2 teaspoons garlic granules
½ teaspoon chilli powder
½ teaspoon dried oregano
¼ teaspoon salt
¼ teaspoon black pepper
5 tomatoes, roughly chopped
1 red pepper, deseeded and
    roughly chopped
2 Scotch bonnet peppers
1 onion, diced
3 tablespoons tomato purée
1 chicken stock cube
½ teaspoon curry powder
½ teaspoon dried oregano
300g (10½oz) long-grain rice
600ml (20fl oz) chicken stock
3 bay leaves

Preheat the oven to 220° fan/475°F/gas mark 9 and line a baking tray with greaseproof paper (or tin foil).

Spray the chicken thighs with a little oil. Mix together the paprika, onion and garlic granules, chilli powder, oregano, salt and pepper and rub over the chicken thighs.

Place the chicken on the baking tray and bake in the oven for 40 minutes.

Meanwhile, place the tomatoes, red pepper and Scotch bonnet peppers in a food processor or blender, and blitz until smooth.

Spray a large saucepan with a little oil and place over a medium-high heat. Add the onions and cook for 6–7 minutes, until golden.

Add the tomato purée, stir, and cook for 2–3 minutes. Add the blended tomato mix and cook for about 30 minutes, stirring frequently.

Reduce the heat to medium and crumble in the stock cube, then add the curry powder and oregano. Stir and cook for 10 minutes, then reduce the heat to low.

Add the rice and stir until everything is well combined, then add the stock and the bay leaves, stir, cover and cook for 30 minutes.

Give the rice a final stir and serve with the chicken.

NOTE

Switch the chillies out for something not so spicy if you aren't a fan!

PERSIAN PROTEIN BOWLS

There's an awful lot going on here for what amounts to a healthy bowl of wonder – our take on a Buddha bowl if you will, and not just because we tend to serve it sat-down, bow-legged with our boobs on show. But look, if you can't be fussed making the tzatziki, just buy ready-made, and you can replace the marinade with a rub. Not that sort of rub, though admittedly you'd burn off a few calories.

SERVES: 4
PREP: 30 minutes
COOK: 40 minutes
CALORIES: 437

6 skinless, boneless chicken
   thighs

For the marinade
1 bunch of fresh coriander,
   finely chopped
2 tablespoons olive oil
1 clove of garlic, crushed or
   grated
1 small green chilli, deseeded
   and finely chopped

For the bowl
6 spring onions, sliced
1 small green chilli, sliced
½ cucumber, deseeded
   and diced
3 tomatoes, chopped
1 red onion, diced
½ bunch of parsley, finely
   chopped
1 tablespoon olive oil
juice of 1 lemon
¼ teaspoon salt
¼ teaspoon black pepper
a pinch of dried chilli flakes
1 tablespoon dried dill
6 cloves of garlic, crushed
   or grated
2 pitta breads

For the tzatziki
400g (14oz) fat-free Greek yoghurt
2 cloves of garlic, crushed or grated
½ teaspoon salt
½ cucumber, deseeded and grated
a handful of mint, chopped
½ teaspoon dried dill

Preheat the oven to 220°C fan/475°F/gas mark 9.

Mix the marinade ingredients together in a small bowl and rub over the chicken thighs, then set aside to marinate for 20 minutes.

Spray a large frying pan with a little oil and place over a medium-high heat. Add the chicken and cook for 5 minutes, then turn and cook for another 5 minutes.

Transfer the chicken to a baking sheet and cook in the oven for 25 minutes, then roughly chop.

Meanwhile, place the spring onions, sliced green chilli, cucumber, tomatoes, red onion and parsley in a bowl. Add the oil, lemon juice, salt, pepper, chilli flakes, dill and garlic, and toss to combine.

Slice the pitta breads in half lengthways (to give 4 'pockets') and bake in the oven for the last 3 minutes of the chicken cooking time.

Mix together the ingredients for the tzatziki.

Serve the chicken with the salad, pitta bread and tzatziki.

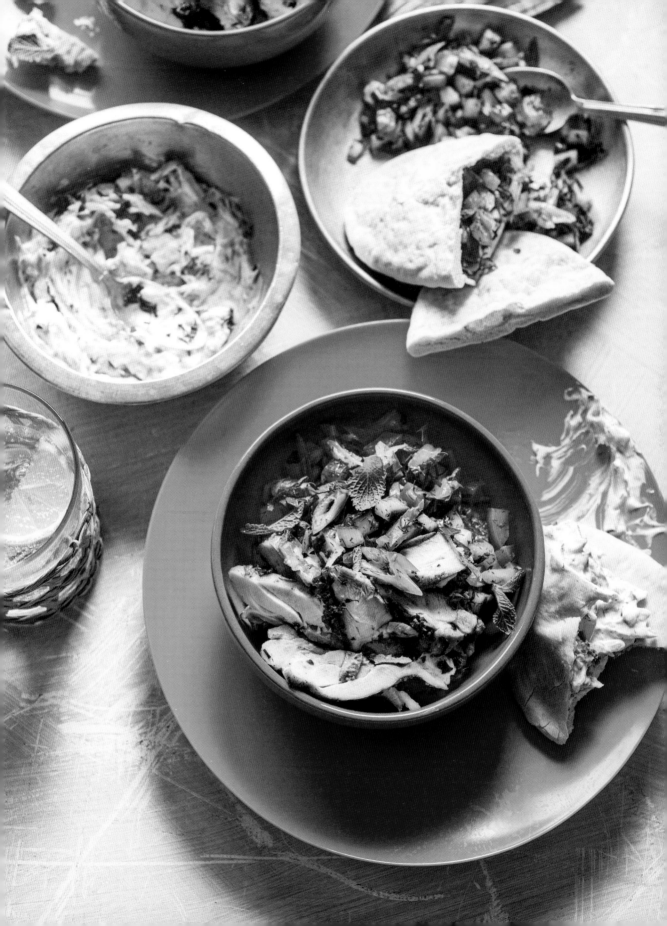

CARAMEL CHICKEN

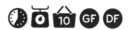

Let's get something out of the way straight off the bat: fish sauce smells like absolute death. If you haven't used it before, consider yourself warned – family members may walk into your kitchen and make the reasonable assumption that you have passed away in front of the hot oven and started rotting. It is putrid. But you must not let such olfactory terrors phase you: it cooks off and leaves a very pleasant taste in this very simple, very plain dish.

Now of course you may look at the sugar here and think we have had a fit of the vapours – and indeed, if you looked in my rucksack those thoughts might carry still more weight – but quite honestly, it's not a great amount and it's worth it for the sticky, golden chicken that awaits. Serve this with some plain rice for a simple, delicious dinner.

SERVES: 4
PREP: 5 minutes
COOK: 40 minutes
CALORIES: 203

6 skinless, boneless chicken thighs
4 cloves of garlic, finely sliced
2 tablespoons fish sauce
¼ teaspoon salt
¼ teaspoon pepper
70g (2½oz) granulated sugar
1 red chilli, sliced

Spray a large frying pan with a little oil and place it on a medium-high heat. Add the chicken and cook for 4–5 minutes on each side, then remove to a plate.

Add the garlic to the pan and cook for 1 minute. Add the fish sauce, salt, pepper and sugar, along with 150ml (5fl oz) of water, and bring to the boil, stirring continuously and scraping the bottom if anything catches.

Return the chicken to the pan, reduce the heat to medium, and cook for 10 minutes. Turn the chicken over, put a lid on the pan, and cook for another 15 minutes, until the sauce thickens and turns a nice caramel colour.

Serve with rice and sprinkle with the red chilli.

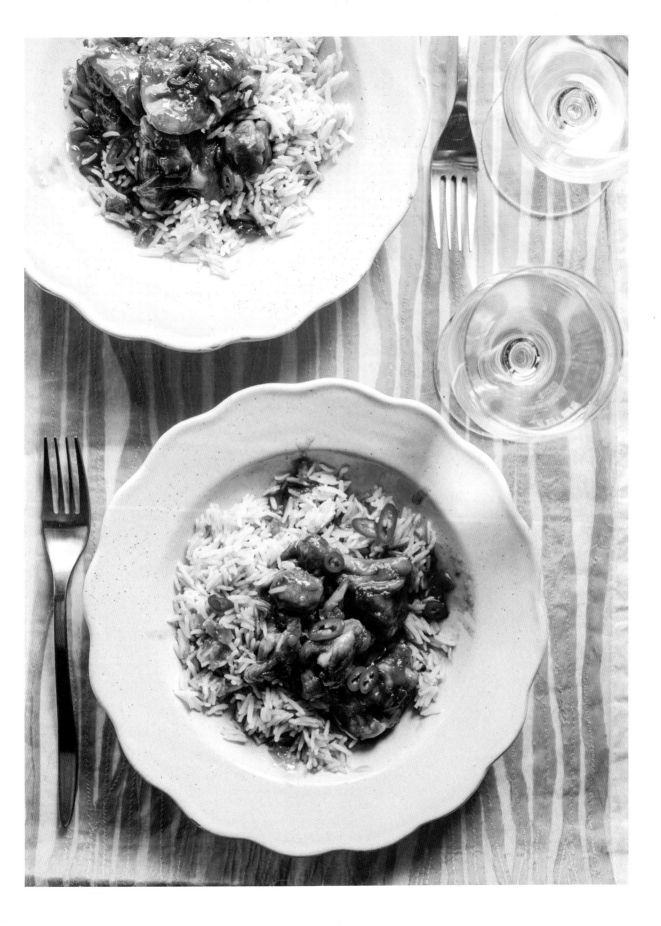

★★★★★ BONUS RECIPE ★★★★★★
CHOCOLATE ORANGE RAINBOW FUDGE

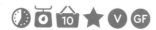

Of course, this isn't a dinner recipe at all, nor is it low in calories. But see, we always try and have one recipe in the books that is rainbow themed and frankly, it doesn't get any brighter than this. This is recipe 101, so we haven't diddled you out of any slimming recipes, before you start hurling bricks through our publisher's doors: this is a little extra bonus. In fact, you could say, we're giving you a happy finish.

Well, look, it was either going to be that or a joke about packing fudge, wasn't it?

This is cheating fudge, mind you – only takes a few ingredients and is very sweet indeed, so eat sparingly. But if you're after something to send your charming little offspring (or even better, someone else's children, mahahaha) to the skies on sugar, this is the ticket.

Do take a second to check the notes before making this! Also, you'll see that we've given the quantities in metric only, as they have to be completely exact for the recipe to work.

MAKES: 45 chunks
PREP: 15 minutes
COOK: at least 8 hours
CALORIES: 180

710g condensed milk
1.1kg white chocolate
gel colourings
chocolate essence
orange essence

NOTES

Oh, look at you following orders – good work!

Try to use a medium straight-edged loaf tin if you can, rather than an angled version. If an angled version is all you can find, fret not, just adjust the layers slightly so you're putting in slightly more as you near the top so the layers are uniform.

We prefer essences to flavourings, as you only need a drop or two for the flavour and adding liquid can be problematic – same with the gels – you only need a drop or two, don't go mad.

Line your loaf tin with foil, taking care to smooth out the wrinkles the best you can and leaving enough hanging over so you can lift it out when it's all done.

Put 118g of condensed milk and 183g of chopped up white chocolate into a microwaveable bowl and microwave in 10-second bursts, stirring like absolute buggery after each. Stop when there are a few lumps left, as the residual heat will take care of the rest.

Add a drop of colouring (the bottom layer, so purple) and a drop of essence (chocolate) and stir.

Gently pour it into your lined loaf tin, being very careful not to drip it on the sides, and then once it has settled, rap the tin a few times on the worktop to get the bubbles out.

Put the tin into the freezer for at least an hour, so there's a skin on the layer, and then repeat the process 5 more times, alternating the flavourings and changing the colour each time.

Once all your layers are done, put it into the fridge overnight.

When it comes to serving, lift it carefully out of the tin using the foil, unwrap it gently, trim off the sides, then slice up, wiping the knife clean every time you cut so the colours don't blend – cheesewire works well too.

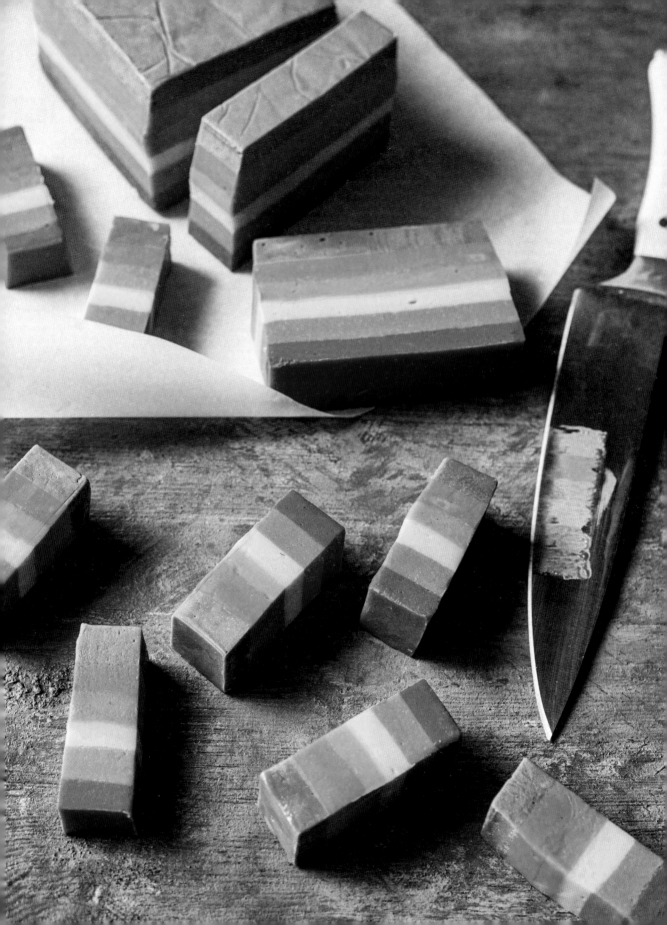

INDEX

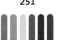

THANK YOU

Traditionally, Paul and I dedicate some lovely words to one another at this point but frankly, there are only so many new things we can say after sixteen years, so, Paul, love, you're brilliant. And, from Paul to James: I'm not one for long messages but you're all right and lovely to cuddle into.

They say romance is dead! In lieu of overwrought panegyrics to one another, we're going to rattle off a list of random acknowledgements in no particular order, but all of significance. Buckle in.

TOGETHER Our fabulous team at Yellow Kite and Hodder, who remain bafflingly invested in our journey. Lauren Whelan, our constant keystone, remains a beautiful ray of sunshine in our group WhatsApp. Isabel Gonzalez-Prendergast, as well as having the most glamorous name in existence (even if it does require me to double-check the spelling), has arrived as our Project Editor and done a sterling job at keeping us smiling and/or writing. Also, excellent GIF work. Clare Skeats has once again taken our words and pictures and made this third book even more vivid and gorgeous than the last.

TOGETHER Our Food Stylists, Photographers and Prop Stylists (Frankie Unsworth, Liz and Max Haarala Hamilton and Jen Kay respectively) have spent days making the food look unbelievably stunning, and honestly, you have no idea how much work goes into this. This book only looks so good because these utterly amazing experts have thrown everything they can at it. Every year we ask for more rainbow and every year they up their game. By book five we'll be expecting actual holograms, although our publishers have nixed our pop-up idea as it'll have someone's eyes out.

JAMES Congratulations to my very best mate Paul 'You're Doing It Wrong' Hawkins (38) (stone), who has managed to clipboard through another year of telling me how I *could* do better if I just *tried* harder and yet somehow made me laugh every single day. Further thanks go to Martin 'Doing It Wrong' Hawkins (38^2), who suffers the pain of his tinnitus ramping up for at least one week per month to allow me to come visit and scatter wet towels upon the floor. Both excellent friends who keep me going in all manner of different ways.

TOGETHER Thank you to our brother from another other, Facebook's Own Gareth Main, who is always there to provide comfort, perspective, laughter and the chance to slip him £10 because he's skint and needs a bottle of Blue Nun and a packet of Sterling to get him through the night.

TOGETHER A personal thank you to our very own Annie Wilkes, Amanda Geisler, because we know it'll absolutely set her away frothing with excitement.

TOGETHER Thank you to Chris, Christine and Deborah for all their support and guidance on how to spend our royalties.

JAMES I have to take a moment to thank Steps for valiantly releasing 112 albums in a single year and soundtracking my journeys, even if they ignored the saladwe named after them. Probably best forgotten.

TOGETHER To every escape room worker who has witnessed Paul and me stumbling around in the dark showing our a*se-cracks every time we bend down.

JAMES I've done a lot of travelling around this year on my lonesome to write, and every B&B I stayed in has been an incredible experience. However, special thanks must go to: Alexandra at Aiden House B&B in Durness (www.aidenhouse.co.uk), Joe, the owner of the beautiful Church House in Scarborough (@churchhousescarborough on Instagram), and Marion and Moray at Applecross B&B (www.applecrossbedandbreakfast.co.uk).

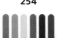

PAUL: Cheers to the regular Fusioners at elite: Cramlington, especially Andrew and Tracey for keeping me motivated and all of the trainers for helping me get fitter – Ben, Benji, Corey, Daryle, Gemma, Lauren and Faye (much missed). You've all helped me more than you know and I'm forever grateful.

TOGETHER Thank you to Tom Owen for his amazing artistic skills and providing us with cheap thrills every time we look at his Instagram @tomowenartist.

PAUL Thank you to the wonderful, ever-fragrant Cyndi who puts up with listening to my bollocks all day. Not literally, they don't make much noise other than a sound like someone peeling cheap ham off a steamy window. She also keeps me caffeinated to the point that it's always a ⁵⁄₀₀ whether I'll kiss any visitors on the lips or punch a hole in the wall.

PAUL Flack and Hill deserve a shout-out for making sure I spend at least five hours a day listening politely to tales of their children, sexual encounters and visits to the clinic. I can put this because I know they're both too tight to actually purchase the book.

JAMES To every single member of the NHS, including my husband: you do the most amazing job in the face of adversity, and although claps won't pay your wages, know that you're appreciated. As someone with health anxiety and a loyalty card for my local GP surgery, I am yet to deal with a single member of staff who hasn't been wonderful. You're badly funded, under-appreciated and the target of mouth-breathers who think watching a YouTube video is the equivalent of understanding medical science, but you carry on regardless – thank you!

TOGETHER Thank you to some of our neighbours for providing endless amusement, and to the better neighbours for being so wonderful when our house burned down, and especially Wilf, Wilma, Colin and Pat, who have kept us in vegetables and a lovely-looking garden all year long.

PAUL Actually, I do just want to take a moment to say thank you to Goomba, who obviously can't read this but I can't let the opportunity to say what a good boy he is pass me by. The Czech writer Milan Kundera wrote that 'dogs are our link to paradise', and he couldn't have been more correct. Coming home to see you waiting for me, your big brown eyes aflame with love and adoration, has made my life sparkle. The moment that James brought you to me, my heart soared and has never floated back to the grey of life before. I promise to be your protector, your guardian, the bringer of food and fun and frolics, new adventures, experiences and wonderful new places. You're my dog, my heart and my everything, and not a moment passes when I don't appreciate how you'll forever shape my life for the better. To my best boy then, you're forever loved, and as a River once said – happy ever after does not mean forever, it just means time. I promise you, my darling dog: our time will be perfect.

JAMES: Cheers babe.

And of course, it almost goes without saying at this point, the biggest thank you goes to you, the reader. You decided to give away your hard-earned money to hopefully find some delightful recipes and wonder how many crude jokes we can make in one sitting. Well, it's a hard one. But looking back over the last two years of success with our books makes us more grateful than ever that we have such a loyal following of funny, clever, smutty, hilarious fans. Without you we'd be two Geordies shouting at each other in the kitchen. You'll never know how much it means to us when we see people cook our recipes, leave us nice comments, take the trouble to leave a review or have a good scrap in our comments. Plus the absolute unadulterated thrill of seeing our book in print out in the wild is still as potent as ever. For all our jokes, cynicism and sarcasm, we love you all.

So, with that, we're off. Happy cooking and toodle-oo.

Endless love and constant pride

James Paul

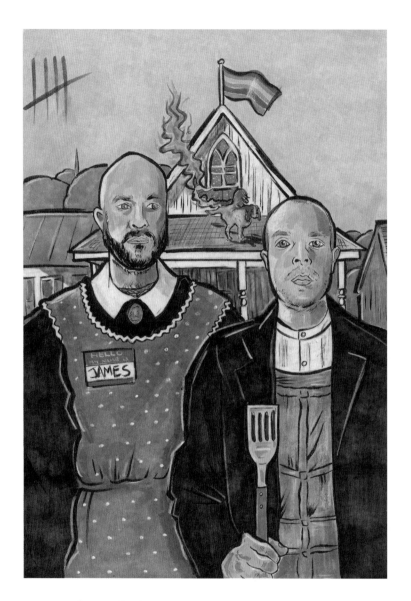

Northern Gothic depicts James and Paul standing in front of their palatial, burning home whilst Goomba attempts to save the day. By local artist and absolute DILF Tom Owen (@tomowenartist).

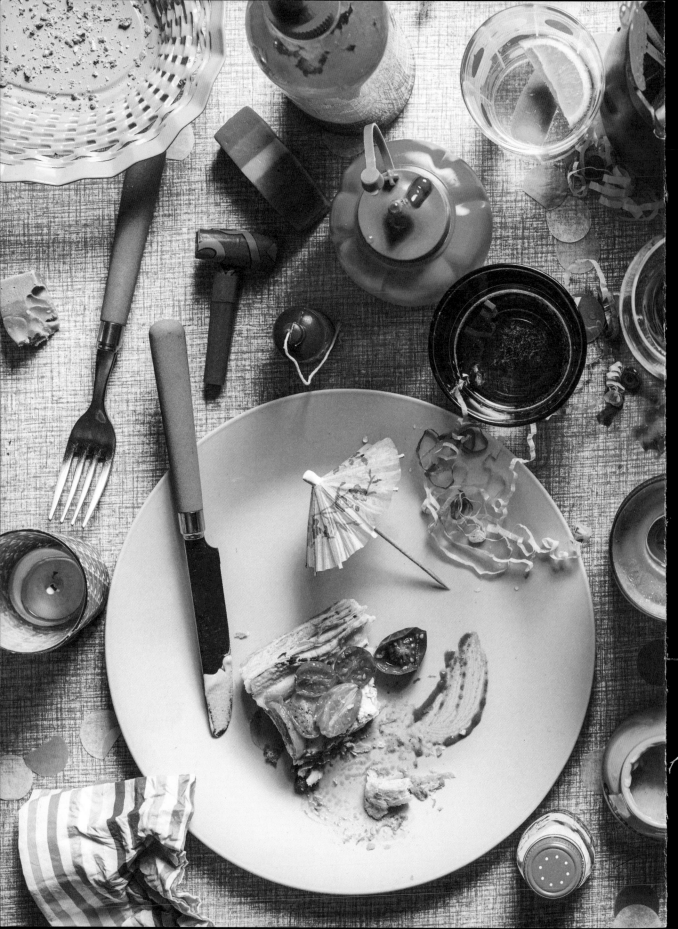